THE LITTLE BOOK FOR GIRLS

M. L. STRATTON

Δadamsmedia

AVON, MASSACHUSETTS

Published by
Adams Media, a division of F+W Media, Inc.
57 Littlefield Street, Avon, MA 02322. U.S.A.
www.adamsmedia.com

ISBN 10: 1-4405-2896-9
ISBN 13: 978-14405-2896-5
eISBN 10: 1-4405-2990-6
eISBN 13: 978-1-4405-2990-0

Printed by RR Donnelley, Harrisonburg, VA, USA.
10 9 8 7 6 5 4 3 2 1
September 2011

Library of Congress Cataloging-in-Publication Data
is available from the publisher.

This publication is designed to provide accurate and authoritative information with regard to the subject matter covered. It is sold with the understanding that the publisher is not engaged in rendering legal, accounting, or other professional advice. If legal advice or other expert assistance is required, the services of a competent professional person should be sought.

— From a *Declaration of Principles* jointly adopted by a Committee of the American Bar Association and a Committee of Publishers and Associations

"A Game of Fives" excerpted from *Phantasmagoria* by Lewis Carroll, London: Macmillan and Co., 1869.

"Good Night and Good Morning" excerpted from *Good Night and Good Morning* by Richard Monckton Milnes, Lord Houghton, Boston: Roberts Brothers, 1883.

"There Was a Little Girl" excerpted from *Random Memories* by Henry Wadsworth Longfellow, Boston: Houghton Mifflin Company, 1922.

"The Three Little Kittens" excerpted from *New Nursery Songs for All Good Children* by Eliza Follen, 1853.

"Here We Go Round the Mulberry Bush" excerpted from *Popular Rhymes and Nursery Tales: A Sequel to The Nursery Rhymes of England* by J. Orchard Halliwell-Phillips, London: John Russell Smith, 1849.

This book is available at quantity discounts for bulk purchases.
For information, please call 1-800-289-0963.

DEDICATION

For my Piper Glory—
the epitome of sugar and spice. *Especially* spice.

❧ ACKNOWLEDGMENTS ❧

Researching and writing this book has been a true joy, and I must begin by wholeheartedly thanking my editor, Andrea, for this wonderful and incredible opportunity. *Thank you.*

And without my amazingly supportive and handsome husband, DBS, I never could have managed such an endeavor. You, I love. My most sincere thanks to my family and my friends for brainstorming with me, for watching my children, for supporting me and encouraging me along the way . . . for everything. I feel so blessed. I can only hope that you, the reader, will enjoy this treasury as much as I've delighted in dreaming it and writing it!

MLS

Matthew 21:16

"If it's half as good as the half we've known, here's Hail! to the rest of the road." Sheldon Vanauken, *A Severe Mercy*

INTRODUCTION

What are little girls made of?
Sugar and spice
And everything nice,
That's what little girls are made of.

No one can steal your heart faster than your darling little girl. Hers is a charm you cannot resist, from her shy smiles and girlish giggles to her pretty pouts and squeals of delight.

There are timeless images that you'll cherish as your beautiful baby girl grows into an even more beautiful young woman: pigtails and pony rides . . . tea parties and teddy bears . . . hopscotch and hugs. Here, in this memorable treasury, you'll find songs, poems, rhymes, and games to share with your daughter to celebrate the things that make being a little girl so special.

Because being special is what being a little girl is all about!

POEMS

Lavender Blue

Lavender's blue, dilly dilly,
Lavender's green
When you are king, dilly dilly,
I shall be queen
Who told you so, dilly dilly,
Who told you so?
'Twas my own heart, dilly dilly,
That told me so
Call up your friends, dilly dilly
Set them to work
Some to the plough, dilly dilly,
Some to the fork
Some to the hay, dilly dilly,
Some to thresh corn
Whilst you and I, dilly dilly,
Keep ourselves warm
Lavender's blue, dilly dilly,
Lavender's green
When you are king, dilly dilly,
I shall be queen
Who told you so, dilly dilly,
Who told you so?
'Twas my own heart, dilly dilly,
That told me so.

Tea and Coffee

Molly, my sister, and I fell out,
And what do you think it was
all about?
She loved coffee and I loved
tea,
And that was the reason we
couldn't agree.

Lucy Locket

Lucy Locket lost her pocket,
Kitty Fisher found it;
There was not a penny in it,
But a ribbon round it.

Little Snow-White

(SNOW WHITE AND THE SEVEN DWARFS)
BY THE BROTHERS GRIMM

t was in the middle of winter, when the broad flakes of snow were falling around, that a certain queen sat working at her window, the frame of which was made of fine black ebony; and, as she was looking out upon the snow, she pricked her finger, and three drops of blood fell upon it. Then she gazed thoughtfully down on the red drops which sprinkled the white snow and said, "Would that my little daughter may be as white as that snow, as red as the blood, and as black as the ebony window-frame!" And so the little girl grew up; her skin was as white as snow, her cheeks as rosy as blood, and her hair as black as ebony; and she was called Snow-White.

But this queen died; and the king soon married another wife, who was very beautiful, but so proud that she could not bear to think that any one could surpass her. She had a magical looking-glass, to which she used to go and gaze upon herself in it, and say—

"Tell me, glass, tell me true!
Of all the ladies in the land,
Who is fairest? Tell me who?"

And the glass answered, "Thou, Queen, art fairest in the land."

But Snow-White grew more and more beautiful; and when she was seven years old, she was as bright as the day, and fairer than the queen herself. Then the glass one day answered the queen, when she went to consult it as usual—

"Thou, Queen, may'st fair and beauteous be,
But Snow-White is lovelier far than thee."

When the queen heard this she turned pale with rage and envy; and calling to one of her servants said, "Take Snow-White away into the wide wood, that I may never see her more." Then the servant led the little girl away; but his heart melted when she begged him to spare her life, and he said, "I will not hurt thee, thou pretty child." So he left her there alone; and though he thought it most likely that the wild beasts would tear her to pieces, he felt as if a great weight were taken off his heart when he had made up his mind not to kill her, but leave her to her fate.

Then poor Snow-White wandered along through the wood in great fear; and the wild beasts roared around, but none did her any harm. In the evening she came to a little cottage, and went in there to rest, for her weary feet would carry her no further. Everything was spruce and neat in the cottage: on the table was spread a white cloth, and there were seven little plates with seven little loaves and seven little glasses with wine in them; and knives and forks laid in order, and by the wall stood seven little beds. Then, as she was exceedingly hungry, she picked a little piece off each loaf, and drank a very little wine out of each glass; and after that she thought she would lie down and rest. So she tried all the little beds; and one was too long, and another was too short, till, at last, the seventh suited her; and there she laid herself down and went to sleep.

Presently in came the masters of the cottage, who were seven little dwarfs that lived among the mountains, and dug and searched about for gold. They lighted up their seven lamps, and saw directly that all was not right. The first said, "Who has been sitting on my stool?" The second, "Who has been eating off my plate?" The third, "Who has been picking at my bread?" The fourth, "Who has been meddling with my spoon?" The fifth, "Who has been handling my fork?" The sixth, "Who has been cutting with my knife?" The seventh, "Who has been drinking my wine?" Then the first looked around and said, "Who has been lying on my bed?" And the rest came running to him, and every one cried out that somebody had been upon his bed. But the seventh saw Snow-White, and called upon his brethren to come and look at her; and they cried out with wonder and astonishment, and brought their lamps and gazing upon her, they said, "Good heavens! what a lovely child she is!" And they were delighted to see her, and took care not to waken her; and the seventh dwarf slept an hour with each of the other dwarfs in turn, till the night was gone.

In the morning Snow-White told them all her story, and they pitied her, and said if she would keep all things in order, and cook and wash, and knit and spin for them, she might stay where she was, and they would take good care of her. Then they went out all day long to their work, seeking for gold and silver in the mountains; and Snow-White remained at home; and they warned her, saying, "The queen will soon find out where you are, so take care and let no one in." But the queen, now that she thought Snow-White was dead, believed that she was certainly the handsomest lady in the land; so she went to her glass and said—

"Tell me, glass, tell me true!
Of all the ladies in the land,
Who is fairest? Tell me who?"
And the glass answered—
"Thou, Queen, thou are fairest in all this land;
But over the Hills, in the greenwood shade,
Where the seven dwarfs their dwelling have made,
There Snow-White is hiding; and she
Is lovelier far, O Queen, than thee."
Then the queen was very much alarmed; for she knew that the glass always spoke the truth, and she was sure that the servant had betrayed her. And as she could not bear to think that any one lived who was more beautiful than she was, she disguised herself as an old pedlar woman and went her way over the hills to the place where the

dwarfs dwelt. Then she knocked at the door and cried, "Fine wares to sell!" Snow-White looked out of the window, and said, "Good day, good woman; what have you to sell?" "Good wares, fine wares," replied she; "laces and bobbins of all colors." "I will let the old lady in; she seems to be a very good sort of a body," thought Snow-White; so she ran down, and unbolted the door. "Bless me!" said the woman, "how badly your stays are laced. Let me lace them up with one of my nice new laces." Snow-White did not dream of any mischief; so she stood up before the old woman who set to work so nimbly, and pulled the lace so tightly that Snow-White lost her breath, and fell down as if she were dead. "There's an end of all thy beauty," said the spiteful queen, and went away home.

In the evening the seven dwarfs returned; and I need not say how grieved they were to see their faithful Snow-White stretched upon the ground motionless, as if she were quite dead. However, they lifted her up, and when they found what was the matter, they cut the lace; and in a little time she began to breathe, and soon came to herself again. Then they said, "The old woman was the queen; take care another time, and let no one in when we are away."

When the queen got home, she went to her glass, and spoke to it, but to her surprise it replied in the same words as before.

Then the blood ran cold in her heart with spite and malice to hear that Snow-White still lived; and she dressed herself up again in a disguise, but very different from the one she wore before, and took with her a poisoned comb. When she reached the dwarfs' cottage, she knocked at the door, and cried, "Fine wares to sell!" but Snow-White said, "I dare not let any one in." Then the queen said, "Only look at my beautiful combs"; and gave her the poisoned one. And it looked so pretty that the little girl took it up and put it into her hair to try it; but the moment it touched her head the poison was so powerful that she fell down senseless. "There you may lie," said the queen, and went her way. But by good luck the dwarfs returned very early that evening; and when they saw Snow-White lying on the ground, they thought what had happened, and soon found the poisoned comb. And when they took it away, she recovered, and told them all that had passed; and they warned her once more not to open the door to any one.

Meantime the queen went home to her glass, and trembled with rage when she received exactly the same answer as before; and she said, "Snow-White shall die, if it costs me my life." So she went secretly into a chamber, and prepared a poisoned apple: the outside looked very rosy and tempting, but whosoever tasted it was sure to die. Then she dressed herself up as a peasant's wife, and traveled over the hills to the dwarfs' cottage, and knocked at the door; but Snow-White put her head out of the window, and said, "I dare not let any one in, for the dwarfs have told me not to." "Do as you please," said the old woman, "but at any rate take this pretty apple; I will make you a present of it." "No," said Snow-White, "I dare not take it." "You silly girl!" answered the other, "what are you afraid of? Do you think it is poisoned? Come! do you eat one part, and I will eat the other."

Now the apple was so prepared that one side was good, though the other side was poisoned. Then Snow-White was very much tempted to taste, for the apple looked exceedingly nice; and when she saw the old woman eat, she could refrain no longer. But she had scarcely put the piece into her mouth when she fell down dead upon the ground. "This time nothing will save thee," said the queen; and she went home to her glass, and at last it said—"Thou, Queen, art the fairest of all the fair." And then her envious heart was glad, and as happy as such a heart could be.

When evening came, and the dwarfs returned home, they found Snow-White lying on the ground; no breath passed her lips, and they were afraid that she was quite dead. They lifted her up, and combed her hair, and washed her face with wine and water; but all was in vain.

So they laid her down upon a bier, and all seven watched and bewailed her three whole days; and then they proposed to bury her; but her cheeks were still rosy, and her face looked just as it did while she was alive; so they said, "We will never bury her in the cold ground." And they made a coffin of glass so that they might still look at her, and wrote her name upon it in golden letters, and that she was a king's daughter. Then the coffin was placed upon the hill, and one of the dwarfs always sat by it and watched. And the birds of the air came, too, and bemoaned Snow-White. First of all came an owl, and then a raven, but at last came a dove.

And thus Snow-White lay for a long, long time, and still only looked as though she were asleep; for she was even now as white as snow, and as red as blood, and as black as ebony. At last a prince came and called at the dwarfs' house; and he saw Snow-White and read what was written in golden letters. Then he offered the dwarfs money, and earnestly prayed them to let him take her away; but they said, "We will not part with her for all the gold in the world." At last, however, they had pity on him, and gave him the coffin; but the moment he lifted it up to carry it home with him, the piece of apple fell from between her lips, and Snow-White awoke, and exclaimed, "Where am I?" And the prince answered, "Thou art safe with me." Then he told her all that had happened, and said, "I love you better than all the world; come with me to my father's palace, and you shall be my wife." Snow-White consented, and went home with the prince; and everything was prepared with great pomp and splendor for their wedding.

To the feast was invited, among the rest, Snow-White's old enemy, the queen; and as she was dressing herself in fine, rich clothes, she looked in the glass and said,

"Tell me, glass, tell me true!
Of all the ladies in the land,
Who is fairest? tell me who?"

And the glass answered,

"Thou, lady, art the loveliest here, I ween;
But lovelier far is the new-made queen."

When she heard this, the queen started with rage; but her envy and curiosity were so great, that she could not help setting out to see the bride. And when she arrived, and saw that it was no other than Snow-White, whom she thought had been dead a long while, she choked with passion, and fell ill and died; but Snow-White and the prince lived and reigned happily over that land, many, many years.

Little girls have a magic all their own.

—Unknown

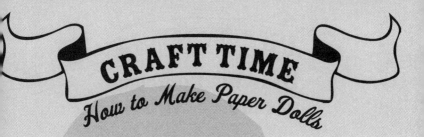

CRAFT TIME
How to Make Paper Dolls

Supplies You'll Need:

- → Construction paper or card stock
- → Pencils to draw doll and accessories
- → Scissors
- → Craft glue
- → Markers, colored pencils, or crayons
- → Old wrapping paper or decorative paper of any sort
- → Ribbon, yarn, old buttons, sequins, stickers, glitter, scraps of cloth

1. Draw a doll pattern on a piece of construction paper (you can use this as a template to make as many dolls as you want, or make different sized patterns to create a doll family!).

2. Carefully cut out the pattern(s) with scissors.

3. Trace around the doll's body on another sheet of paper (wrapping, decorative, or construction paper) in the shape of clothes for your doll. Don't forget to make tabs on the clothes to fold over the doll's body!

4. Use the ribbon, sequins, etc. to decorate your clothes. You can also create accessories like purses, shoes, and jewelry.

HERE WE GO ROUND
THE MULBERRY BUSH

Here we go round the
mulberry bush

The mulberry bush, the
mulberry bush

Here we go round the
mulberry bush

So early in the morning

This is the way we wash
our clothes

Wash our clothes, wash
our clothes

This is the way we wash
our clothes

So early Monday morning

This is the way we iron
our clothes

Iron our clothes, iron
our clothes

This is the way we iron
our clothes

So early Tuesday morning

This is the way we mend
our clothes

Mend our clothes, mend
our clothes

This is the way we mend
our clothes

So early Wednesday morning

This is the way we sweep
the floor

Sweep the floor, sweep
the floor

This is the way we sweep
the floor

So early Thursday morning

This is the way we
scrub the floor

Scrub the floor, scrub the floor

This is the way we scrub
the floor

So early Friday morning

This is the way we bake
our bread

Bake our bread, bake our bread

This is the way we bake
our bread

So early Saturday morning

This is the way we go to church

Go to church, go to church

This is the way we go
to church

So early Sunday morning

Like stardust glistening on fairies' wings, little girls' dreams are of magical things.

—SHERRY LARSON

POEMS

Round and Round the Garden

Round and Round the garden
Round and round the garden
Like a teddy bear.
One step, two step,
Tickle you under there

One Two, Buckle My Shoe

One, two, buckle my shoe;
Three, four, knock at the door;
Five, six, pick up sticks;
Seven, eight, lay them straight;
Nine, ten, a good, fat hen;
Eleven, twelve, dig and delve;
Thirteen, fourteen, maids a-
courting;
Fifteen, sixteen, maids in the
kitchen;
Seventeen, eighteen, maids a-
waiting;
Nineteen, twenty, my plate's
empty.

The Queen of Hearts

The Queen of Hearts,
She made some tarts
all on a summer's day;
The Knave of Hearts,
He stole those tarts,
And took them clean away.
The King of Hearts
Called for the tarts
And beat the Knave full sore;
The Knave of Hearts
Brought back the tarts,
And vowed he'd steal no more.

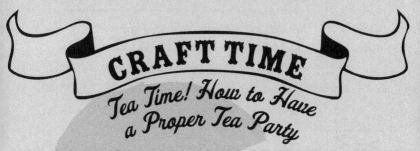

CRAFT TIME

Tea Time! How to Have a Proper Tea Party

- ↔ *Who:* You, your daughter, some friends or dolls
- ↔ *What:* A Proper Tea
- ↔ *When:* Anytime between 3:30 P.M. and 5:00 P.M.
- ↔ *Where:* In the garden (don't forget your hat!), in the dining room . . . any charming and comfortable spot
- ↔ *Why:* For fun!

Here's how:

The basics: You'll need a teapot, teacups and saucers, a sugar bowl (or sugar cubes), lemon, a creamer for milk, serving plates for your fare, knives for spreading, teaspoons for stirring, and forks if you're serving cake.

Setting the table: Make the table as beautiful and as fancy as you like. Linen tablecloths and napkins are a must, but don't worry about all of your china or linens matching.

Things to serve: Cookies, scones, cakes, jam, tea sandwiches, biscuits, muffins, crumpets, tortes.

How to serve: First comes tea, served by the hostess, who asks the guests how they would like their tea prepared. The hostess adds the accompaniments to each cup and the guests stir. When everyone has been served, the savory foods, like sandwiches, are passed. When plates are empty, it's on to the bread course, where items like scones and muffins are served. And after the bread course is finished, it's time to bring out the cakes and cookies and begin the dessert course. Bon appétit!

Little Thumbelina

BY HANS CHRISTIAN ANDERSEN

here was once a woman who wished very much to have a little child. She went to a fairy and said: "I should so very much like to have a little child. Can you tell me where I can find one?"

"Oh, that can be easily managed," said the fairy. "Here is a barleycorn; it is not exactly of the same sort as those which grow in the farmers' fields, and which the chickens eat. Put it into a flowerpot and see what will happen."

"Thank you," said the woman; and she gave the fairy twelve shillings, which was the price of the barleycorn. Then she went home and planted it, and there grew up a large, handsome flower, somewhat like a tulip in appearance, but with its leaves tightly closed, as if it were still a bud.

"It is a beautiful flower," said the woman, and she kissed the red and golden-colored petals; and as she did so the flower opened, and she could see that it was a real tulip. But within the flower, upon the green velvet stamens, sat a very delicate and graceful little maiden. She was scarcely half as long as a thumb, and they gave her the name of Little Thumb, or Thumbelina, because she was so small.

A walnut shell, elegantly polished, served her for a cradle; her bed was formed of blue violet leaves, with a rose leaf for a counterpane. Here she slept at night, but during the day she amused herself on a table, where the peasant wife had placed a plate full of water.

Round this plate were wreaths of flowers with their stems in the water, and upon it floated a large tulip leaf, which served the little one for a boat. Here she sat and rowed herself from side to side, with two oars made of white horsehair. It was a very pretty sight. Thumbelina could also sing so softly and sweetly that nothing like her singing had ever before been heard.

One night, while she lay in her pretty bed, a large, ugly, wet toad crept through a broken pane of glass in the window and leaped right upon the table where she lay sleeping under her rose-leaf quilt.

"What a pretty little wife this would make for my son," said the toad, and she took up the walnut shell in which Thumbelina lay asleep, and jumped through the window with it, into the garden.

In the swampy margin of a broad stream in the garden lived the toad with her son. He was uglier even than his mother; and when he saw the pretty little maiden in her elegant bed, he could only cry "Croak, croak, croak."

"Don't speak so loud, or she will wake," said the toad, "and then she might run away, for she is as light as swan's-down. We will place her on one of the water-lily leaves out in the stream; it will be like an island to her, she is so light and small, and then she cannot escape; and while she is there we will make haste and prepare the stateroom under the marsh, in which you are to live when you are married."

Far out in the stream grew a number of water lilies with broad green leaves which seemed to float on the top of the water. The largest of these leaves appeared farther off than the rest, and the old toad swam out to it with the walnut shell, in which Thumbelina still lay asleep.

The tiny creature woke very early in the morning and began to cry bitterly when she found where she was, for she could see nothing but water on every side of the large green leaf, and no way of reaching the land.

Meanwhile the old toad was very busy under the marsh, decking her room with rushes and yellow wildflowers, to make it look pretty for her new daughter-in-law. Then she swam out with her ugly son to the leaf on which she had placed poor Thumbelina. She wanted to bring the pretty bed, that she might put it in the bridal chamber to be ready for her. The old toad bowed low to her in the water and said, "Here is my son; he will be your husband, and you will live happily together in the marsh by the stream."

"Croak, croak, croak," was all her son could say for himself. So the toad took up the elegant little bed and swam away with it, leaving Thumbelina all alone on the green leaf, where she sat and wept. She could not bear to think of living with the old toad and having her ugly son for a husband. The little fishes who swam about in the water beneath had seen the toad and heard what she said, so now they lifted their heads above the water to look at the little maiden.

As soon as they caught sight of her they saw she was very pretty, and it vexed them to think that she must go and live with the ugly toads.

"No, it must never be!" So they gathered together in the water, round the green stalk which held the leaf on which the little maiden stood, and gnawed it away at the root with their teeth. Then the leaf floated down the stream, carrying Thumbelina far away out of reach of land.

Thumbelina sailed past many towns, and the little birds in the bushes saw her and sang, "What a lovely little creature." So the leaf swam away with her farther and farther, till it brought her to other lands. A graceful little white butterfly constantly fluttered round her and at last alighted on the leaf. The little maiden pleased him, and she was glad of it, for now the toad could not possibly reach her, and the country through which she sailed was beautiful, and the sun shone upon the water till it glittered like liquid gold. She took off her girdle and tied one end of it round the butterfly, fastening the other end of the ribbon to the leaf, which now glided on much faster than before, taking Thumbelina with it as she stood.

Presently a large cockchafer flew by. The moment he caught sight of her he seized her round her delicate waist with his claws and flew with her into a tree. The green leaf floated away on the brook, and the butterfly flew with it, for he was fastened to it and could not get away.

Oh, how frightened Thumbelina felt when the cockchafer flew with her to the tree! But especially was she sorry for the beautiful white butterfly which she had fastened to the leaf, for if he could not free himself he would die of hunger. But the cockchafer did not trouble himself at all about the matter. He seated himself by her side, on a large green leaf, gave her some honey from the flowers to eat, and told her she was very pretty, though not in the least like a cockchafer.

After a time all the cockchafers who lived in the tree came to pay Thumbelina a visit. They stared at her, and then the young lady cockchafers turned up their feelers and said, "She has only two legs! how ugly that looks." "She has no feelers," said another. "Her waist is quite slim. Pooh! she is like a human being."

"Oh, she is ugly," said all the lady cockchafers. The cockchafer who had run away with her believed all the others when they said she was ugly. He would have nothing more to say to her, and told her she might go where she liked. Then he flew down with her from the tree and placed her on a daisy, and she wept at the thought that she was so ugly that even the cockchafers would have nothing to say to her. And all the while she was really the loveliest creature that one could imagine, and as tender and delicate as a beautiful rose leaf.

During the whole summer poor little Thumbelina lived quite alone in the wide forest. She wove herself a bed with blades of grass and hung it up under a broad leaf, to protect herself from the rain. She sucked the honey from the flowers for food and drank the dew from their leaves every morning.

So passed away the summer and the autumn, and then came the winter—the long, cold winter. All the birds who had sung to her so sweetly had flown away, and the trees and the flowers had withered. The large shamrock under the shelter of which she had lived was now rolled together and shriveled up; nothing remained but a yellow, withered stalk. She felt dreadfully cold, for her clothes were torn, and she was herself so frail and delicate that she was nearly frozen to death. It began to snow, too; and the snowflakes, as they fell upon her, were like a whole shovelful falling upon one of us, for we are tall, but she was only an inch high. She wrapped herself in a dry leaf, but it cracked in the middle and could not keep her warm, and she shivered with cold.

Near the wood in which she had been living was a large cornfield, but the corn had been cut a long time; nothing remained but the bare, dry stubble, standing up out of the frozen ground. It was to her like struggling through a large wood.

Oh! how she shivered with the cold. She came at last to the door of a field mouse, who had a little den under the corn stubble. There dwelt the field mouse in warmth and comfort, with a whole roomful of corn, a kitchen, and a beautiful dining room. Poor Thumbelina stood before the door, just like a little beggar girl, and asked for a small piece of barleycorn, for she had been without a morsel to eat for two days.

"You poor little creature," said the field mouse, for she was really a good old mouse, "come into my warm room and dine with me."

She was pleased with Thumbelina, so she said, "You are quite welcome to stay with me all the winter, if you like; but you must keep my rooms clean and neat, and tell me stories, for I shall like to hear them very much." And Thumbelina did all that the field mouse asked her, and found herself very comfortable.

"We shall have a visitor soon," said the field mouse one day; "my neighbor pays me a visit once a week. He is better off than I am; he has large rooms, and wears a beautiful black velvet coat. If you could only have him for a husband, you would be well provided for indeed. But he is blind, so you must tell him some of your prettiest stories."

Thumbelina did not feel at all interested about this neighbor, for he was a mole. However, he came and paid his visit, dressed in his black velvet coat.

"He is very rich and learned, and his house is twenty times larger than mine," said the field mouse.

He was rich and learned, no doubt, but he always spoke slightingly of the sun and the pretty flowers, because he had never seen them. Thumbelina was obliged to sing to him, "Ladybird, ladybird, fly away home," and many other pretty songs. And the mole fell in love with her because she had so sweet a voice; but he said nothing yet, for he was very prudent and cautious. A short time before, the mole had dug a long passage under the earth, which led from the dwelling of the field mouse to his own, and here she had permission to walk with Thumbelina whenever she liked. But he warned them not to be alarmed at the sight of a dead bird which lay in the passage. It was a perfect bird, with a beak and feathers, and could not have been dead long. It was lying just where the mole had made his passage. The mole took in his mouth a piece of phosphorescent wood, which glittered like fire in the dark. Then he went before them to light them through the long, dark passage. When they came to the spot where the dead bird lay, the mole pushed his broad nose through the ceiling, so that the earth gave way and the daylight shone into the passage.

In the middle of the floor lay a swallow, his beautiful wings pulled close to his sides, his feet and head drawn up under his feathers — the poor bird had evidently died of the cold. It made little Thumbelina very sad to see it, she did so love the little birds; all the summer they had sung and twittered for her so beautifully. But the mole pushed it aside with his crooked legs and said: "He will sing no more now. How miserable it must be to be born a little bird! I am thankful that none of my children will ever be birds, for they can do nothing but cry 'Tweet, tweet,' and must always die of hunger in the winter."

"Yes, you may well say that, as a clever man!" exclaimed the field mouse. "What is the use of his twittering if, when winter comes, he must either starve or be frozen to death? Still, birds are very high bred."

Thumbelina said nothing, but when the two others had turned their backs upon the bird, she stooped down and stroked aside the soft feathers which covered his head, and kissed the closed eyelids. "Perhaps this was the one who sang to me so sweetly in the summer," she said; "and how much pleasure it gave me, you dear, pretty bird."

The mole now stopped up the hole through which the daylight shone, and then accompanied the ladies home. But during the night Thumbelina could not sleep; so she got out of bed and wove a large, beautiful carpet of hay. She carried it to the dead bird and spread it over him, with some down from the flowers which she had found in the field mouse's room. It was as soft as wool, and she spread some of it on each side of the bird, so that he might lie warmly in the cold earth.

"Farewell, pretty little bird," said she, "farewell. Thank you for your delightful singing during the summer, when all the trees were green and the warm sun shone upon us." Then she laid her head on the bird's breast, but she was alarmed, for it seemed as if something inside the bird went "thump, thump." It was the bird's heart; he was not really dead, only benumbed with the cold, and the warmth had restored him to life. In autumn all the swallows fly away into warm countries; but if one happens to linger, the cold seizes it, and it becomes chilled and falls down as if dead. It remains where it fell, and the cold snow covers it.

Thumbelina trembled very much; she was quite frightened, for the bird was large, a great deal larger than herself (she was only an inch high). But she took courage, laid the wool more thickly over the poor swallow, and then took a leaf which she had used for her own counterpane and laid it over his head.

The next night she again stole out to see him. He was alive, but very weak; he could only open his eyes for a moment to look at Thumbelina, who stood by, holding a piece of decayed wood in her hand, for she had no other lantern. "Thank you, pretty little maiden," said the sick swallow; "I have been so nicely warmed that I shall soon regain my strength and be able to fly about again in the warm sunshine."

"Oh," said she, "it is cold out of doors now; it snows and freezes. Stay in your warm bed; I will take care of you."

She brought the swallow some water in a flower leaf, and after he had drunk, he told her that he had wounded one of his wings in a thornbush and could not fly as fast as the others, who were soon far away on their journey to warm countries. At last he had fallen to the earth, and could remember nothing more, nor how he came to be where she had found him.

All winter the swallow remained underground, and Thumbelina nursed him with care and love. She did not tell either the mole or the field mouse anything about it, for they did not like swallows. Very soon the springtime came, and the sun warmed the earth. Then the swallow bade farewell to Thumbelina, and she opened the hole in the ceiling which the mole had made. The sun shone in upon them so beautifully that the swallow asked her if she would go with him. She could sit on his back, he said, and he would fly away with her into the green woods. But she knew it would grieve the field mouse if she left her in that manner, so she said, "No, I cannot."

"Farewell, then, farewell, you good, pretty little maiden," said the swallow, and he flew out into the sunshine.

Thumbelina looked after him, and the tears rose in her eyes. She was very fond of the poor swallow.

"Tweet, tweet," sang the bird, as he flew out into the green woods, and Thumbelina felt very sad. She was not allowed to go out into the warm sunshine. The corn which had been sowed in the field over the house of the field mouse had grown up high into the air and formed a thick wood to Thumbelina, who was only an inch in height.

"You are going to be married, little one," said the field mouse. "My neighbor has asked for you. What good fortune for a poor child like you! Now we will prepare your wedding clothes. They must be woolen and linen. Nothing must be wanting when you are the wife of the mole."

Thumbelina had to turn the spindle, and the field mouse hired four spiders, who were to weave day and night. Every evening the mole visited her and was continually speaking of the time when the summer would be over. Then he would keep his wedding day with Thumbelina; but now the heat of the sun was so great that it burned the earth and made it hard, like stone. As soon as the summer was over the wedding should take place. But Thumbelina was not at all pleased, for she did not like the tiresome mole.

Every morning when the sun rose and every evening when it went down she would creep out at the door, and as the wind blew aside the ears of corn so that she could see the blue sky, she thought how beautiful and bright it seemed out there and wished so much to see her dear friend, the swallow, again. But he never returned, for by this time he had flown far away into the lovely green forest.

When autumn arrived Thumbelina had her outfit quite ready, and the field mouse said to her, "In four weeks the wedding must take place."

Then she wept and said she would not marry the disagreeable mole.

"Nonsense," replied the field mouse. "Now don't be obstinate, or I shall bite you with my white teeth. He is a very handsome mole; the queen herself does not wear more beautiful velvets and furs. His kitchens and cellars are quite full. You ought to be very thankful for such good fortune."

So the wedding day was fixed, on which the mole was to take her away to live with him, deep under the earth, and never again to see the warm sun, because *he* did not like it. The poor child was very unhappy at the thought of saying farewell to the beautiful sun, and as the field mouse had given her permission to stand at the door, she went to look at it once more.

"Farewell, bright sun," she cried, stretching out her arm towards it; and then she walked a short distance from the house, for the corn had been cut, and only the dry stubble remained in the fields. "Farewell, farewell," she repeated, twining her arm around a little red flower that grew just by her side. "Greet the little swallow from me, if you should see him again."

"Tweet, tweet," sounded over her head suddenly. She looked up, and there was the swallow himself flying close by. As soon as he spied Thumbelina he was delighted. She told him how unwilling she was to marry the ugly mole, and to live always beneath the earth, nevermore to see the bright sun. And as she told him, she wept.

"Cold winter is coming," said the swallow, "and I am going to fly away into warmer countries. Will you go with me? You can sit on my back and fasten yourself on with your sash. Then we can fly away from the ugly mole and his gloomy rooms—far away, over the mountains, into warmer countries, where the sun shines more brightly than here; where it is always summer, and the flowers bloom in greater beauty. Fly now with me, dear little one; you saved my life when I lay frozen in that dark, dreary passage."

"Yes, I will go with you," said Thumbelina; and she seated herself on the bird's back, with her feet on his outstretched wings, and tied her girdle to one of his strongest feathers.

The swallow rose in the air and flew over forest and over sea—high above the highest mountains, covered with eternal snow.

Thumbelina would have been frozen in the cold air, but she crept under the bird's warm feathers, keeping her little head uncovered, so that she might admire the beautiful lands over which they passed. At length they reached the warm countries, where the sun shines brightly and the sky seems so much higher above the earth. Here on the hedges and by the wayside grew purple, green, and white grapes, lemons and oranges hung from trees in the fields, and the air was fragrant with myrtles and orange blossoms. Beautiful children ran along the country lanes, playing with large gay butterflies; and as the swallow flew farther and farther, every place appeared still more lovely.

At last they came to a blue lake, and by the side of it, shaded by trees of the deepest green, stood a palace of dazzling white marble, built in the olden times. Vines clustered round its lofty pillars, and at the top were many swallows' nests, and one of these was the home of the swallow who carried Thumbelina.

"This is my house," said the swallow; "but it would not do for you to live there—you would not be comfortable. You must choose for yourself one of those lovely flowers, and I will put you down upon it, and then you shall have everything that you can wish to make you happy."

"That will be delightful," she said, and clapped her little hands for joy.

A large marble pillar lay on the ground, which, in falling, had been broken into three pieces. Between these pieces grew the most beautiful large white flowers, so the swallow flew down with Thumbelina and placed her on one of the broad leaves. But how surprised she was to see in the middle of the flower a tiny little man, as white and transparent as if he had been made of crystal! He had a gold crown on his head, and delicate wings at his shoulders, and was not much larger than was she herself. He was the angel of the flower, for a tiny man and a tiny woman dwell in every flower, and this was the king of them all.

"Oh, how beautiful he is!" whispered Thumbelina to the swallow.

The little prince was at first quite frightened at the bird, who was like a giant compared to such a delicate little creature as himself; but when he saw Thumbelina he was delighted and thought her the prettiest little maiden he had ever seen. He took the gold crown from his head and placed it on hers, and asked her name and if she would be his wife and queen over all the flowers.

This certainly was a very different sort of husband from the son of the toad, or the mole with his black velvet and fur, so she said Yes to the handsome prince. Then all the flowers opened, and out of each came a little lady or a tiny lord, all so pretty it was quite a pleasure to look at them. Each of them brought Thumbelina a present; but the best gift was a pair of beautiful wings, which had belonged to a large white fly, and they fastened them to Thumbelina's shoulders, so that she might fly from flower to flower.

Then there was much rejoicing, and the little swallow, who sat above them in his nest, was asked to sing a wedding song, which he did as well as he could; but in his heart he felt sad, for he was very fond of Thumbelina and would have liked never to part from her again.

"You must not be called Thumbelina any more," said the spirit of the flowers to her. "It is an ugly name, and you are so very lovely. We will call you Maia."

"Farewell, farewell," said the swallow, with a heavy heart, as he left the warm countries, to fly back into Denmark. There he had a nest over the window of a house in which dwelt the writer of fairy tales. The swallow sang "Tweet, tweet," and from his song came the whole story.

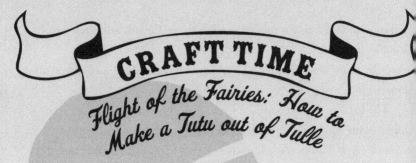

CRAFT TIME

Flight of the Fairies: How to Make a Tutu out of Tulle

Little girls love to dress up, and this simple-to-make fairy tutu will have your daughter twirling and dancing with delight!

What You'll Need:

- 5 to 20 yards of 6" tulle, depending on how full and how long you want your tutu to be
- 18 to 24" of ribbon for the waistband (1 to 2" wired ribbon will work best)

1. Decide how long you want your tutu to be. Measure the length from the waist and then double that number.

2. With sharp scissors, cut your tulle into strips measuring the length you arrived at in the first step, and as wide as you like. Narrower strips will be easier to tie onto the waistband.

3. Lay out the long ribbon piece that will be the waistband. Fold a strip of tulle in half across the middle and lay it on top of the waistband, in the middle of the ribbon. Loop the fold around the waistband and slip the loose ends of the tulle through the loop, making a slipknot around the waistband. Secure the tulle onto the ribbon by tightening the slipknot.

4. Continue attaching the strips of tulle to the ribbon waistband in this way until there is enough tulle attached to make a full skirt (the closer you tie on the strips of tulle, the fuller the skirt will be). Then simply wrap it around your little girl's waist and tie the excess wired ribbon into a bow.

A toddling little girl is a centre of common feeling which makes the most dissimilar people understand each other.

——GEORGE ELIOT

Hansel and Gretel

BY THE BROTHERS GRIMM

ard by a great forest dwelt a poor wood-cutter with his wife and his two children. The boy was called Hansel and the girl Gretel. He had little to bite and to break, and once when great dearth fell on the land, he could no longer procure even daily bread. Now when he thought over this by night in his bed, and tossed about in his anxiety, he groaned and said to his wife: "What is to become of us? How are we to feed our poor children, when we no longer have anything even for ourselves?" "I'll tell you what, husband, answered the woman, early to-morrow morning we will take the children out into the forest to where it is the thickest; there we will light a fire for them, and give each of them one more piece of bread, and then we will go to our work and leave them alone. They will not find the way home again, and we shall be rid of them." "No, wife," said the man, "I will not do that. How can I bear to leave my children alone in the forest? —the wild animals would soon come and tear them to pieces." "O, you fool," said she, then we must all four die of hunger, you may as well plane the planks for our coffins," and she left him no peace until he consented. "But I feel very sorry for the poor children, all the same," said the man.

The two children had also not been able to sleep for hunger, and had heard what their step-mother had said to their father. Gretel wept bitter tears, and said to Hansel: "Now all is over with us." "Be quiet, Gretel," said Hansel, "do not distress yourself, I will soon find a way to help us." And when the old folks had fallen asleep, he got up, put on his little coat, opened the door below, and crept outside. The moon shone brightly, and the white pebbles which lay in front of the house glittered like real silver pennies. Hansel stooped and stuffed the little pocket of his coat with as many as he could get in. Then he went back and said to Gretel: "Be comforted, dear little sister, and sleep in peace, God will not forsake us," and he lay down again in his bed.

When day dawned, but before the sun had risen, the woman came and awoke the two children, saying: "Get up, you sluggards! we are going into the forest to fetch wood." She gave each a little piece of bread, and said, "There is something for your dinner, but do not eat it up before then, for you will get nothing else." Gretel took the bread under her apron, as Hansel had the pebbles in his pocket. Then they all set out together on the way to the forest. When they had walked a short time, Hansel stood still and peeped back at the house, and did so again and again. His father said: "Hansel, what are you looking at there and staying behind for? Pay attention, and do not forget how to use your legs." "Ah, father," said Hansel, "I am looking at my little white cat, which is sitting up on the roof, and wants to say good-bye to me." The wife said, "Fool, that is not your little cat, that is the morning sun which is shining on the chimneys." Hansel, however, had not been looking back at the cat, but had been constantly throwing one of the white pebble-stones out of his pocket on the road.

When they had reached the middle of the forest, the father said: "Now, children, pile up some wood, and I will light a fire that you may not be cold." Hansel and Gretel gathered brushwood together, as high as a little hill. The brushwood was lighted, and when the flames were burning very high, the woman said: "Now, children, lay yourselves down by the fire and rest, we will go into the forest and cut some wood. When we have done, we will come back and fetch you away."

Hansel and Gretel sat by the fire, and when noon came, each ate a little piece of bread, and as they heard the strokes of the wood-axe they believed that their father was near. It was not the axe, however, but a branch which he had fastened to a withered tree which the wind was blowing backwards and forwards. And as they had been sitting such a long time, their eyes closed with fatigue, and they fell fast asleep. When at last they awoke, it was already dark night. Gretel began to cry and said, "How are we to get out of the forest now?" But Hansel comforted her and said: "Just wait a little, until the moon has risen, and then we will soon find the way." And when the full moon had risen, Hansel took his little sister by the hand, and followed the pebbles which shone like newly-coined silver pieces, and showed them the way.

They walked the whole night long, and by break of day came once more to their father's house. They knocked at the door, and when the woman opened it and saw that it was Hansel and Gretel, she said: "You naughty children, why have you slept so long in the forest? —we thought you were never coming back at all!" The father, however, rejoiced, for it had cut him to the heart to leave them behind alone.

Not long afterwards, there was once more great dearth throughout the land, and the children heard their mother saying at night to their father: "Everything is eaten again, we have one half loaf left, and that is the end. The children must go, we will take them farther into the wood, so that they will not find their way out again; there is no other means of saving ourselves!" The man's heart was heavy, and he thought: "It would be better for you to share the last mouthful with your children." The woman, however, would listen to nothing that he had to say, but scolded and reproached him. He who says A must say B, likewise, and as he had yielded the first time, he had to do so a second time also.

The children, however, were still awake and had heard the conversation. When the old folks were asleep, Hansel again got up, and wanted to go out and pick up pebbles as he had done before, but the woman had locked the door, and Hansel could not get out. Nevertheless he comforted his little sister, and said, "Do not cry, Gretel, go to sleep quietly, the good God will help us."

Early in the morning came the woman, and took the children out of their beds. Their piece of bread was given to them, but it was still smaller than the time before. On the way into the forest Hansel crumbled his in his pocket, and often stood still and threw a morsel on the ground. "Hansel, why do you stop and look round?" said the father, "go on." "I am looking back at my little pigeon which is sitting on the roof, and wants to say good-bye to me," answered Hansel. "Fool," said the woman, "that is not your little pigeon, that is the morning sun that is shining on the chimney." Hansel, however, little by little, threw all the crumbs on the path.

The woman led the children still deeper into the forest, where they had never in their lives been before. Then a great fire was again made, and the mother said, "Just sit there, you children, and when you are tired you may sleep a little; we are going into the forest to cut wood, and in the evening when we are done, we will come and fetch you away." When it was noon, Gretel shared her piece of bread with Hansel, who had scattered his by the way. Then they fell asleep and evening passed, but no one came to the poor children. They did not awake until it was dark night, and Hansel comforted his little sister and said, "Just wait, Gretel, until the moon rises, and then we shall see the crumbs of bread which I have strewn about, they will show us our way home again." When the moon came they set out, but they found no crumbs, for the many thousands of birds which fly about in the woods and fields had picked them all up. Hansel said to Gretel: "We shall soon find the way," but they did not find it. They walked the whole night and all the next day too from morning till evening, but they did not get out of the forest, and were very hungry, for they had nothing to eat but two or three berries, which grew on the ground. And as they were so weary that their legs would carry them no longer, they lay down beneath a tree and fell asleep.

It was now three mornings since they had left their father's house. They began to walk again, but they always came deeper into the forest, and if help did not come soon, they must die of hunger and weariness. When it was mid-day, they saw a beautiful snow-white bird sitting on a bough, which sang so delightfully that they stood still and listened to it. And when its song was over, it spread its wings and flew away before them, and they followed it until they reached a little house, on the roof of which it alighted. And when they approached the little house they saw that it was built of bread and covered with cakes, but that the windows were of clear sugar. "We will set to work on that," said Hansel, "and have a good meal. I will eat a bit of the roof, and you Gretel, can eat some of the window, it will taste sweet." Hansel reached up above, and broke off a little of the roof to try how it tasted, and Gretel leant against the window and nibbled at the panes. Then a soft voice cried from the parlor:

"Nibble, nibble, gnaw,

Who is nibbling at my little house?"

The children answered:

"The wind, the wind,

The heaven-born wind,"

and went on eating without disturbing themselves. Hansel, who liked the taste of the roof, tore down a great piece of it, and Gretel pushed out the whole of one round window-pane, sat down, and enjoyed herself with it. Suddenly the door opened, and a woman as old as the hills, who supported herself on crutches, came creeping out. Hansel and Gretel were so terribly frightened that they let fall what they had in their hands. The old woman, however, nodded her head, and said: "Oh, you dear children, who has brought you here? Do come in, and stay with me. No harm shall happen to you." She took them both by the hand, and led them into her little house. Then good food was set before them, milk and pancakes, with sugar, apples, and nuts. Afterwards two pretty little beds were covered with clean white linen, and Hansel and Gretel lay down in them, and thought they were in heaven.

The old woman had only pretended to be so kind; she was in reality a wicked witch, who lay in wait for children, and had only built the little house of bread in order to entice them there. When a child fell into her power, she killed it, cooked and ate it, and that was a feast day with her. Witches have red eyes, and cannot see far, but they have a keen scent like the beasts, and are aware when human beings draw near. When Hansel and Gretel came into her neighborhood, she laughed with malice, and said mockingly: "I have them, they shall not escape me again!"

Early in the morning before the children were awake, she was already up, and when she saw both of them sleeping and looking so pretty, with their plump and rosy cheeks, she muttered to herself: "That will be a dainty mouthful." Then she seized Hansel with her shriveled hand, carried him into a little stable, and locked him in behind a grated door. Scream as he might, it would not help him. Then she went to Gretel, shook her till she awoke, and cried: "Get up, lazy thing, fetch some water, and cook something good for your brother, he is in the stable outside, and is to be made fat. When he is fat, I will eat him." Gretel began to weep bitterly, but it was all in vain, for she was forced to do what the wicked witch commanded.

And now the best food was cooked for poor Hansel, but Gretel got nothing but crab-shells. Every morning the woman crept to the little stable, and cried: "Hansel, stretch out your finger that I may feel if you will soon be fat." Hansel, however, stretched out a little bone to her, and the old woman, who had dim eyes, could not see it, and thought it was Hansel's finger, and was astonished that there was no way of fattening him. When four weeks had gone by, and Hansel still remained thin, she was seized with impatience and would not wait any longer. "Now, then, Gretel," she cried to the girl, "stir yourself, and bring some water. Let Hansel be fat or lean, to-morrow I will kill him, and cook him." Ah, how the poor little sister did lament when she had to fetch the water, and how her tears did flow down her cheeks! "Dear God, do help us," she cried. "If the wild beasts in the forest had but devoured us, we should at any rate have died together." "Just keep your noise to yourself," said the old woman, "it won't help you at all."

Early in the morning, Gretel had to go out and hang up the cauldron with the water, and light the fire. "We will bake first," said the old woman, "I have already heated the oven, and kneaded the dough." She pushed poor Gretel out to the oven, from which flames of fire were already darting. "Creep in," said the witch, and see if it properly heated, so that we can put the bread in." And once Gretel was inside, she intended to shut the oven and let her bake in it, and then she would eat her, too. But Gretel saw what she had in mind, and said: "I do not know how I am to do it; how do I get in?" "Silly goose," said the old woman. "The door is big enough; just look, I can get in myself!" and she crept up and thrust her head into the oven. Then Gretel gave her a push that drove her far into it, and shut the iron door, and fastened the bolt. Oh! then she began to howl quite horribly, but Gretel ran away, and the godless witch was miserably burnt to death.

Gretel, however, ran like lightning to Hansel, opened his little stable, and cried: "Hansel, we are saved! The old witch is dead!" Then Hansel sprang like a bird from its cage when the door is opened. How they did rejoice and embrace each other, and dance about and kiss each other! And as they had no longer any need to fear her, they went into the witch's house, and in every corner there stood chests full of pearls and jewels. "These are far better than pebbles!" said Hansel, and thrust into his pockets whatever could be got in, and Gretel said: "I, too, will take something home with me," and filled her pinafore full. "But now we must be off," said Hansel, "that we may get out of the witch's forest."

When they had walked for two hours, they came to a great stretch of water. "We cannot cross," said Hansel, "I see no foot-plank, and no bridge." "And there is also no ferry," answered Gretel, "but a white duck is swimming there; if I ask her, she will help us over." Then she cried:

"Little duck, little duck, dost thou see,

Hansel and Gretel are waiting for thee.

There's never a plank, nor bridge in sight,

Take us across on thy back so white."

The duck came to them, and Hansel seated himself on its back, and told his sister to sit by him. "No," replied Gretel, "that will be too heavy for the little duck; she shall take us across, one after the other." The good little duck did so, and when they were once safely across and had walked for a short time, the forest seemed to be more and more familiar to them, and at length they saw from afar their father's house. Then they began to run, rushed into the parlor, and threw themselves round their father's neck. The man had not known one happy hour since he had left the children in the forest; the woman, however, was dead. Gretel emptied her pinafore until pearls and precious stones ran about the room, and Hansel threw one handful after another out of his pocket to add to them. Then all anxiety was at an end, and they lived together in perfect happiness. My tale is done, there runs a mouse, whosoever catches it, may make himself a big fur cap out of it.

LET THE GOOD TIMES ROLL

If you need a little mother/daughter or father/daughter time, here are a few suggestions that your little girl will love!

- Share an ice cream sundae
- Play dolls together
- Find a new playground
- Dress up
- Have a tea party
- Read a book
- Snuggle
- Paint her fingernails
- Take a class together
- Be silly
- Play hairdresser
- Go to the movies
- Fly a kite
- Play a sport
- Dance!
- Play a board game
- Take a walk
- Make a sand castle
- Use your imagination
- Do a craft
- Explore
- Tickle and tackle
- Explore the zoo
- Sing songs
- Race!
- Cook a meal
- Bake a treat
- Volunteer
- Paint each other's portrait
- Pick flowers
- Make holiday decorations
- Play a card game
- Do a puzzle
- Visit a friend
- Make a card
- Go see a play
- Play tag
- Make up stories
- Go to the museum
- Have a spa day
- Hula hoop!
- Read poetry
- Learn how to latch hook
- Have a puppet show
- Paint each other's faces
- Tell knock-knock jokes
- Make jewelry
- Play a card game

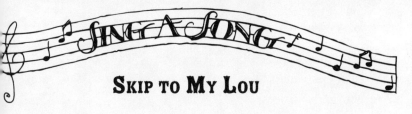

SKIP TO MY LOU

Lou, Lou, skip to my Lou
Lou, Lou, skip to my Lou
Lou, Lou, skip to my Lou
Skip to my Lou, my darlin'!
Fly's in the buttermilk,
Shoo, fly, shoo,
Fly's in the buttermilk,
Shoo, fly, shoo,
Fly's in the buttermilk,
Shoo, fly, shoo,
Skip to my Lou, my darlin'.
Lou, Lou, skip to my Lou
Lou, Lou, skip to my Lou
Lou, Lou, skip to my Lou
Skip to my Lou, my darlin'!
Lost my partner,
What'll I do?
Lost my partner,
What'll I do?

Lost my partner,
What'll I do?
Skip to my Lou, my darlin'.
Lou, Lou, skip to my Lou
Lou, Lou, skip to my Lou
Lou, Lou, skip to my Lou
Skip to my Lou, my darlin'!
I'll find another one,
Prettier, too,
I'll find another one,
Prettier, too,
I'll find another one,
Prettier, too,
Skip to my Lou, my darlin'.

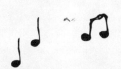
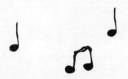

To a father growing old
nothing is dearer than
a daughter.

——EURIPIDES

CLASSIC FATHER-DAUGHTER MOVIES

- *Curly Sue*
- *Annie*
- *Father of the Bride*
- *Three Men and a Little Lady*
- *Cheaper by the Dozen*
- *The Game Plan*
- *Daddy's Little Girls*
- *Pride and Prejudice*
- *I Am Sam*
- *Definitely, Maybe*
- *A Tree Grows in Brooklyn*
- *Flicka*
- *Grace Is Gone*
- *On Golden Pond*
- *The Little Princess*

CLASSIC MOTHER-DAUGHTER MOVIES

- *Freaky Friday*
- *The Sound of Music*
- *Terms of Endearment*
- *The Joy Luck Club*
- *Anywhere But Here*
- *Stepmom*
- *Steel Magnolias*
- *Where the Heart Is*
- *Fried Green Tomatoes*
- *Beaches*
- *Driving Miss Daisy*
- *Guarding Tess*
- *How to Make an American Quilt*
- *Chocolat*

GAMES TO PLAY WITH YOUR LITTLE GIRL

- Cat's Cradle
- Marbles
- Pick-up Sticks
- Hide-and-Seek
- Patty-Cake
- Jump Rope
- Foursquare
- Duck, Duck, Goose
- Red Light, Green Light
- Follow the Leader
- Stop and Go
- Simon Says
- Hot Potato
- Freeze Tag

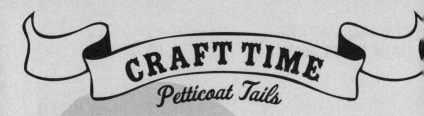

CRAFT TIME
Petticoat Tails

Petticoat Tails are rumored to get their name from the French chefs that worked for Mary Queen of Scots. They called the cookies they made for her *Petit Gautelles,* or "little cakes." This was Anglicized by the Scots, and we know them as Petticoat Tails.

Ingredients

YIELDS 60 COOKIES

- 1 cup unsalted butter
- 1 cup confectioners' sugar
- 1 teaspoon vanilla
- 2½ cups all-purpose flour
- ¼ teaspoon salt

1. Cream together butter, confectioners' sugar, and vanilla. Blend in flour and salt. Wrap; chill overnight.

2. Preheat oven to 400°F.

3. Roll teaspoons of dough into balls; place 2" apart on cookie sheets.

4. Press down with the bottom of a glass dipped in sugar until cookies are ⅛" thick.

5. Bake 8–10 minutes, or until lightly browned.

POEMS

Minnie and Winnie

BY ALFRED,
LORD TENNYSON

Minnie and Winnie
Slept in a shell.
Sleep, little ladies!
And they slept well.
Pink was the shell within,
Silver without;
Sounds of the great sea
Wandered about.
Sleep, little ladies!
Wake not soon!
Echo on echo
Dies to the moon.
Two bright stars
Peeped into the shell.
"What are you dreaming of?
Who can tell?"
Started a green linnet
Out of the croft;
Wake, little ladies,
The sun is aloft!

The Cat and the Fiddle

Hey, diddle, diddle,
The cat and the fiddle,
The cow jumped over the moon;
The little dog laughed to
see such sport,
And the dish ran away
with the spoon.

A-Tisket, A-Tasket

A-tisket, a-tasket,
A green and yellow basket.
I wrote a letter to my love,
But on the way I dropped it.
I dropped it, I dropped it,
And, on the way I dropped it.
A little boy picked it up,
And put it in his pocket.

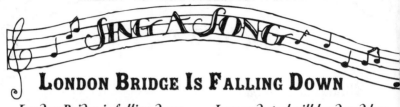

LONDON BRIDGE IS FALLING DOWN

London Bridge is falling down,
Falling down, falling down.
London Bridge is falling down,
My fair lady.

Build it up with wood and clay,
Wood and clay, wood and clay,
Build it up with wood and clay,
My fair lady.

Wood and clay will wash away,
Wash away, wash away,
Wood and clay will wash away,
My fair lady.

Build it up with bricks and mortar,
Bricks and mortar, bricks and
mortar,
Build it up with bricks and mortar,
My fair lady.

Bricks and mortar will not stay,
Will not stay, will not stay,
Bricks and mortar will not stay,
My fair lady.

Build it up with iron and steel,
Iron and steel, iron and steel,
Build it up with iron and steel,
My fair lady.

Iron and steel will bend and bow,
Bend and bow, bend and bow,
Iron and steel will bend and bow,
My fair lady.

Build it up with silver and gold,
Silver and gold, silver and gold,
Build it up with silver and gold,
My fair lady.

Silver and gold will be stolen away,
Stolen away, stolen away,
Silver and gold will be stolen away,
My fair lady.

Set a man to watch all night,
Watch all night, watch all night,
Set a man to watch all night,
My fair lady.

Suppose the man should fall asleep,
Fall asleep, fall asleep,
Suppose the man should fall
asleep?
My fair lady.

Give him a pipe to smoke all night,
Smoke all night, smoke all night,
Give him a pipe to smoke all night,
My fair lady.

The Ugly Duckling

BY HANS CHRISTIAN ANDERSEN

t was so beautiful in the country. It was the summer time. The wheat fields were golden, the oats were green, and the hay stood in great stacks in the green meadows. The stork paraded about among them on his long red legs, chattering away in Egyptian, the language he had learned from his lady mother.

All around the meadows and cornfields grew thick woods, and in the midst of the forest was a deep lake. Yes, it was beautiful, it was delightful in the country.

In a sunny spot stood a pleasant old farmhouse circled all about with deep canals; and from the walls down to the water's edge grew great burdocks, so high that under the tallest of them a little child might stand upright. The spot was as wild as if it had been in the very center of the thick wood.

In this snug retreat sat a duck upon her nest, watching for her young brood to hatch; but the pleasure she had felt at first was almost gone; she had begun to think it a wearisome task, for the little ones were so long coming out of their shells, and she seldom had visitors. The other ducks liked much better to swim about in the canals than to climb the slippery banks and sit under the burdock leaves to have a gossip with her. It was a long time to stay so much by herself.

At length, however, one shell cracked, and soon another, and from each came a living creature that lifted its head and cried "Peep, peep."

"Quack, quack!"said the mother; and then they all tried to say it, too, as well as they could, while they looked all about them on every side at the tall green leaves. Their mother allowed them to look about as much as they liked, because green is good for the eyes.

"What a great world it is, to be sure," said the little ones, when they found how much more room they had than when they were in the eggshell.

"Is this all the world, do you imagine?" said the mother. "Wait till you have seen the garden. Far beyond that it stretches down to the pastor's field, though I have never ventured to such a distance. Are you all out?" she continued, rising to look. "No, not all; the largest egg lies there yet, I declare. I wonder how long this business is to last. I'm really beginning to be tired of it;" but for all that she sat down again.

"Well, and how are you to-day?" quacked an old duck who came to pay her a visit.

"There's one egg that takes a deal of hatching. The shell is hard and will not break," said the fond mother, who sat still upon her nest. "But just look at the others. Have I not a pretty family? Are they not the prettiest little ducklings you ever saw? They are the image of their father—the good for naught! He never comes to see me."

"Let me see the egg that will not break," said the old duck. "I've no doubt it's a Guinea fowl's egg. The same thing happened to me once, and a deal of trouble it gave me, for the young ones are afraid of the water. I quacked and clucked, but all to no purpose. Let me take a look at it. Yes, I am right; it's a Guinea fowl, upon my word; so take my advice and leave it where it is. Come to the water and teach the other children to swim."

"I think I will sit a little while longer," said the mother. "I have sat so long, a day or two more won't matter."

"Very well, please yourself," said the old duck, rising; and she went away.

At last the great egg broke, and the latest bird cried "Peep, peep," as he crept forth from the shell. How big and ugly he was! The mother duck stared at him and did not know what to think. "Really," she said, "this is an enormous duckling, and it is not at all like any of the others. I wonder if he will turn out to be a Guinea fowl. Well, we shall see when we get to the water—for into the water he must go, even if I have to push him in myself."

On the next day the weather was delightful. The sun shone brightly on the green burdock leaves, and the mother duck took her whole family down to the water and jumped in with a splash. "Quack, quack!" cried she, and one after another the little ducklings jumped in. The water closed over their heads, but they came up again in an instant and swam about quite prettily, with their legs paddling under them as easily as possible; their legs went of their own accord; and the ugly gray-coat was also in the water, swimming with them.

"Oh," said the mother, "that is not a Guinea fowl. See how well he uses his legs, and how erect he holds himself! He is my own child, and he is not so very ugly after all, if you look at him properly. Quack, quack! come with me now. I will take you into grand society and introduce you to the farmyard, but you must keep close to me or you may be trodden upon; and, above all, beware of the cat."

When they reached the farmyard, there was a wretched riot going on; two families were fighting for an eel's head, which, after all, was carried off by the cat. "See, children, that is the way of the world," said the mother duck, whetting her beak, for she would have liked the eel's head herself. "Come, now, use your legs, and let me see how well you can behave. You must bow your heads prettily to that old duck yonder; she is the highest born of them all and has Spanish blood; therefore she is well off. Don't you see she has a red rag tied to her leg, which is something very grand and a great honor for a duck; it shows that every one is anxious not to lose her, and that she is to be noticed by both man and beast. Come, now, don't turn in your toes; a well-bred duckling spreads his feet wide apart, just like his father and mother, in this way; now bend your necks and say 'Quack!'"

The ducklings did as they were bade, but the other ducks stared, and said, "Look, here comes another brood—as if there were not enough of us already! And bless me, what a queer-looking object one of them is; we don't want him here"; and then one flew out and bit him in the neck.

"Let him alone," said the mother; "he is not doing any harm."

"Yes, but he is so big and ugly. He's a perfect fright," said the spiteful duck, "and therefore he must be turned out. A little biting will do him good."

"The others are very pretty children," said the old duck with the rag on her leg, "all but that one. I wish his mother could smooth him up a bit; he is really ill-favored."

"That is impossible, your grace," replied the mother. "He is not pretty, but he has a very good disposition and swims as well as the others or even better. I think he will grow up pretty, and perhaps be smaller. He has remained too long in the egg, and therefore his figure is not properly formed;" and then she stroked his neck and smoothed the feathers, saying: "It is a drake, and therefore not of so much consequence. I think he will grow up strong and able to take care of himself."

"The other ducklings are graceful enough," said the old duck. "Now make yourself at home, and if you find an eel's head you can bring it to me."

And so they made themselves comfortable; but the poor duckling who had crept out of his shell last of all and looked so ugly was bitten and pushed and made fun of, not only by the ducks but by all the poultry.

"He is too big," they all said; and the turkey cock, who had been born into the world with spurs and fancied himself really an emperor, puffed himself out like a vessel in full sail and flew at the duckling. He became quite red in the head with passion, so that the poor little thing did not know where to go, and was quite miserable because he was so ugly as to be laughed at by the whole farmyard.

So it went on from day to day; it got worse and worse. The poor duckling was driven about by every one; even his brothers and sisters were unkind to him and would say, "Ah, you ugly creature, I wish the cat would get you" and his mother had been heard to say she wished he had never been born. The ducks pecked him, the chickens beat him, and the girl who fed the poultry pushed him with her feet. So at last he ran away, frightening the little birds in the hedge as he flew over the palings. "They are afraid because I am so ugly," he said. So he flew still farther, until he came out on a large moor inhabited by wild ducks. Here he remained the whole night, feeling very sorrowful.

In the morning, when the wild ducks rose in the air, they stared at their new comrade. "What sort of a duck are you?" they all said, coming round him.

He bowed to them and was as polite as he could be, but he did not reply to their question. "You are exceedingly ugly," said the wild ducks; "but that will not matter if you do not want to marry one of our family."

Poor thing! he had no thoughts of marriage; all he wanted was permission to lie among the rushes and drink some of the water on the moor. After he had been on the moor two days, there came two wild geese, or rather goslings, for they had not been out of the egg long, which accounts for their impertinence. "Listen, friend," said one of them to the duckling; "you are so ugly that we like you very well. Will you go with us and become a bird of passage? Not far from here is another moor, in which there are some wild geese, all of them unmarried. It is a chance for you to get a wife. You may make your fortune, ugly as you are."

"Bang, bang," sounded in the air, and the two wild geese fell dead among the rushes, and the water was tinged with blood. "Bang, bang," echoed far and wide in the distance, and whole flocks of wild geese rose up from the rushes.

The sound continued from every direction, for the sportsmen surrounded the moor, and some were even seated on branches of trees, overlooking the rushes. The blue smoke from the guns rose like clouds over the dark trees, and as it floated away across the water, a number of sporting dogs bounded in among the rushes, which bent beneath them wherever they went. How they terrified the poor duckling! He turned away his head to hide it under his wing, and at the same moment a large, terrible dog passed quite near him. His jaws were open, his tongue hung from his mouth, and his eyes glared fearfully. He thrust his nose close to the duckling, showing his sharp teeth, and then "splash, splash," he went into the water, without touching him.

"Oh," sighed the duckling, "how thankful I am for being so ugly; even a dog will not bite me."

And so he lay quite still, while the shot rattled through the rushes, and gun after gun was fired over him. It was late in the day before all became quiet, but even then the poor young thing did not dare to move. He waited quietly for several hours and then, after looking carefully around him, hastened away from the moor as fast as he could. He ran over field and meadow till a storm arose, and he could hardly struggle against it.

Towards evening he reached a poor little cottage that seemed ready to fall, and only seemed to remain standing because it could not decide on which side to fall first. The storm continued so violent that the duckling could go no farther. He sat down by the cottage, and then he noticed that the door was not quite closed, in consequence of one of the hinges having given way. There was, therefore, a narrow opening near the bottom large enough for him to slip through, which he did very quietly, and got a shelter for the night. Here, in this cottage, lived a woman, a cat, and a hen. The cat, whom his mistress called "My little son," was a great favorite; he could raise his back, and purr, and could even throw out sparks from his fur if it were stroked the wrong way. The hen had very short legs, so she was called "Chickie Short-legs." She laid good eggs, and her mistress loved her as if she had been her own child. In the morning the strange visitor was discovered; the cat began to purr and the hen to cluck.

"What is that noise about?" said the old woman, looking around the room. But her sight was not very good; therefore when she saw the duckling she thought it must be a fat duck that had strayed from home. "Oh, what a prize!" she exclaimed. "I hope it is not a drake, for then I shall have some ducks' eggs. I must wait and see."

So the duckling was allowed to remain on trial for three weeks; but there were no eggs.

Now the cat was the master of the house, and the hen was the mistress; and they always said, "We and the world," for they believed themselves to be half the world, and by far the better half, too. The duckling thought that others might hold a different opinion on the subject, but the hen would not listen to such doubts.

"Can you lay eggs?" she asked. "No." "Then have the goodness to cease talking." "Can you raise your back, or purr, or throw out sparks?" said the cat. "No." "Then you have no right to express an opinion when sensible people are speaking." So the duckling sat in a corner, feeling very low-spirited; but when the sunshine and the fresh air came into the room through the open door, he began to feel such a great longing for a swim that he could not help speaking of it.

"What an absurd idea!" said the hen. "You have nothing else to do; therefore you have foolish fancies. If you could purr or lay eggs, they would pass away."

"But it is so delightful to swim about on the water," said the duckling, "and so refreshing to feel it close over your head while you dive down to the bottom."

"Delightful, indeed! it must be a queer sort of pleasure," said the hen. "Why, you must be crazy! Ask the cat—he is the cleverest animal I know; ask him how he would like to swim about on the water, or to dive under it, for I will not speak of my own opinion. Ask our mistress, the old woman; there is no one in the world more clever than she is. Do you think she would relish swimming and letting the water close over her head?"

"I see you don't understand me," said the duckling.

"We don't understand you? Who can understand you, I wonder? Do you consider yourself more clever than the cat or the old woman?—I will say nothing of myself. Don't imagine such nonsense, child, and thank your good fortune that you have been so well received here. Are you not in a warm room and in society from which you may learn something? But you are a chatterer, and your company is not very agreeable. Believe me, I speak only for your good. I may tell you unpleasant truths, but that is a proof of my friendship. I advise you, therefore, to lay eggs and learn to purr as quickly as possible."

"I believe I must go out into the world again," said the duckling.

"Yes, do," said the hen. So the duckling left the cottage and soon found water on which it could swim and dive, but he was avoided by all other animals because of his ugly appearance.

Autumn came, and the leaves in the forest turned to orange and gold; then, as winter approached, the wind caught them as they fell and whirled them into the cold air. The clouds, heavy with hail and snowflakes, hung low in the sky, and the raven stood among the reeds, crying, "Croak, croak." It made one shiver with cold to look at him. All this was very sad for the poor little duckling.

One evening, just as the sun was setting amid radiant clouds, there came a large flock of beautiful birds out of the bushes. The duckling had never seen any like them before. They were swans; and they curved their graceful necks, while their soft plumage shone with dazzling whiteness. They uttered a singular cry as they spread their glorious wings and flew away from those cold regions to warmer countries across the sea. They mounted higher and higher in the air, and the ugly little duckling had a strange sensation as he watched them. He whirled himself in the water like a wheel, stretched out his neck towards them, and uttered a cry so strange that it frightened even himself. Could he ever forget those beautiful, happy birds! And when at last they were out of his sight, he dived under the water and rose again almost beside himself with excitement. He knew not the names of these birds nor where they had flown, but he felt towards them as he had never felt towards any other bird in the world.

He was not envious of these beautiful creatures; it never occurred to him to wish to be as lovely as they. Poor ugly creature, how gladly he would have lived even with the ducks, had they only treated him kindly and given him encouragement.

The winter grew colder and colder; he was obliged to swim about on the water to keep it from freezing, but every night the space on which he swam became smaller and smaller. At length it froze so hard that the ice in the water crackled as he moved, and the duckling had to paddle with his legs as well as he could, to keep the space from closing up. He became exhausted at last and lay still and helpless, frozen fast in the ice.

Early in the morning a peasant who was passing by saw what had happened. He broke the ice in pieces with his wooden shoe and carried the duckling home to his wife. The warmth revived the poor little creature; but when the children wanted to play with him, the duckling thought they would do him some harm, so he started up in terror, fluttered into the milk pan, and splashed the milk about the room. Then the woman clapped her hands, which frightened him still more. He flew first into the butter cask, then into the meal tub and out again. What a condition he was in! The woman screamed and struck at him with the tongs; the children laughed and screamed and tumbled over each other in their efforts to catch him, but luckily he escaped. The door stood open; the poor creature could just manage to slip out among the bushes and lie down quite exhausted in the newly fallen snow.

It would be very sad were I to relate all the misery and privations which the poor little duckling endured during the hard winter; but when it had passed he found himself lying one morning in a moor, amongst the rushes. He felt the warm sun shining and heard the lark singing and saw that all around was beautiful spring.

Then the young bird felt that his wings were strong, as he flapped them against his sides and rose high into the air. They bore him onwards until, before he well knew how it had happened, he found himself in a large garden. The apple trees were in full blossom, and the fragrant elders bent their long green branches down to the stream, which wound round a smooth lawn. Everything looked beautiful in the freshness of early spring. From a thicket close by came three beautiful white swans, rustling their feathers and swimming lightly over the smooth water. The duckling saw these lovely birds and felt more strangely unhappy than ever.

"I will fly to these royal birds," he exclaimed, "and they will kill me because, ugly as I am, I dare to approach them. But it does not matter; better be killed by them than pecked by the ducks, beaten by the hens, pushed about by the maiden who feeds the poultry, or starved with hunger in the winter."

Then he flew to the water and swam towards the beautiful swans. The moment they espied the stranger they rushed to meet him with outstretched wings.

"Kill me," said the poor bird and he bent his head down to the surface of the water and awaited death.

But what did he see in the clear stream below? His own image — no longer a dark-gray bird, ugly and disagreeable to look at, but a graceful and beautiful swan.

To be born in a duck's nest in a farmyard is of no consequence to a bird if it is hatched from a swan's egg. He now felt glad at having suffered sorrow and trouble, because it enabled him to enjoy so much better all the pleasure and happiness around him; for the great swans swam round the newcomer and stroked his neck with their beaks, as a welcome.

Into the garden presently came some little children and threw bread and cake into the water.

"See," cried the youngest, "there is a new one;" and the rest were delighted, and ran to their father and mother, dancing and clapping their hands and shouting joyously, "There is another swan come; a new one has arrived."

Then they threw more bread and cake into the water and said, "The new one is the most beautiful of all, he is so young and pretty." And the old swans bowed their heads before him.

Then he felt quite ashamed and hid his head under his wing, for he did not know what to do, he was so happy — yet he was not at all proud. He had been persecuted and despised for his ugliness, and now he heard them say he was the most beautiful of all the birds. Even the elder tree bent down its boughs into the water before him, and the sun shone warm and bright. Then he rustled his feathers, curved his slender neck, and cried joyfully, from the depths of his heart, "I never dreamed of such happiness as this while I was the despised ugly duckling."

Be to her virtues very kind, be to her faults a little blind.

——MATTHEW PRIOR

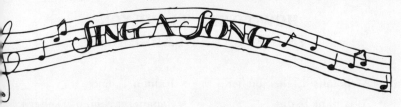
TWINKLE, TWINKLE, LITTLE STAR

Twinkle, twinkle, little star,
How I wonder what you are!
Up above the world so high,
Like a diamond in the sky!
Twinkle, twinkle, little star,
How I wonder what you are!
When the blazing sun is gone,
When the nothing shines upon,
Then you show your little light,
Twinkle, twinkle, all the night.
Twinkle, twinkle, little star,
How I wonder what you are!
Then the traveler in the dark,
Thanks you for your tiny spark,
He could not see which way to go,
If you did not twinkle so.
Twinkle, twinkle, little star,
How I wonder what you are!
In the dark blue sky you keep,
And often through my
  curtains peep,
For you never shut your eye,
Till the sun is in the sky.
Twinkle, twinkle, little star,
How I wonder what you are!
As your bright and tiny spark,
Lights the traveler in the dark, —
Though I know not what you are,
Twinkle, twinkle, little star.

POLLY, PUT THE KETTLE ON

Polly, put the kettle on,
Polly, put the kettle on,
Polly, put the kettle on,
We'll all have tea.
Sukey, take it off again,
Sukey, take it off again,
Sukey, take it off again,
They've all gone away.

HOW TO SAY "I LOVE YOU" IN DIFFERENT LANGUAGES

- **Afrikaans:** Ek het jou lief
- **Albanian:** Te dua
- **Armenian:** Yes kez si'rumem
- **Cantonese:** Ngo oi ney
- **Creole:** Mi aime jou
- **Danish:** Jeg elsker dig
- **Dutch:** Ik hou van jou
- **English:** I love you
- **Filipino:** Iniibig kita
- **Finnish:** Mina rakastan sinua
- **French:** Je t'aime
- **German:** Ich liebe dich
- **Greek:** S'agapo
- **Hawaiian:** Aloha wau ia 'oe
- **Hungarian:** Szeretlek te'ged
- **Icelandic:** Eg elska thig
- **Indonesian:** Saya cinta padamu
- **Irish/Gaelic:** Taim i' ngra leat
- **Italian:** Ti amo
- **Japanese:** Kimi o ai shiteru
- **Korean:** Dangsinul sarang-hee yo
- **Malaysian:** Saya cinta mu
- **Mandarin:** Wo ay ni
- **Norwegian:** Jeg elsker deg
- **Polish:** Kocham cie
- **Portuguese (Brazilian):** Eu te amo
- **Romanian:** Te iubesc
- **Russian:** Ya lyublyu tyebya
- **Spanish:** Te amo
- **Swahili:** Nakupenda
- **Swedish:** Jag älskar dig
- **Ukrainian:** Ya tebe kokhaju
- **Vietnamese:** Toi yeu em

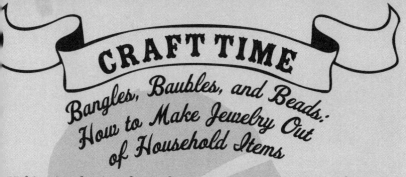

CRAFT TIME

Bangles, Baubles, and Beads: How to Make Jewelry Out of Household Items

Making jewelry is a fun and creative activity to enjoy with your daughter. You can make adorable jewelry with everyday items. Below are some ideas to get you started making unique pieces together!

Materials to use:

- Hollow uncooked pasta noodles (such as macaroni)
- Buttons
- Pieces of candy or cereal
- Beads
- Soda can tabs
- Old keys
- Bottle caps
- Pieces of old or broken jewelry
- Small tiles
- Trinkets or charms
- Safety pins
- Shells and sea glass
- Washers, grommets, small hardware pieces
- Small toys
- Pieces of felt
- Drinking straws
- Dried clay or dough
- Chain
- Rope (like bakers' twine)
- Twine
- Ribbon
- Gimp
- Wire
- Thread (and a needle)
- Shoelaces
- Elastic
- Raffia

To string your jewelry:

- Strips of cloth
- String
- Yarn
- Leather cord

To Get You Started:

You could use markers to color different dry pasta noodles, then string them all up with a piece of fun-colored yarn. Try using a piece of ribbon and some washers to make a jingle-jangle bracelet. Take a plastic sewing needle and a piece or two of string licorice to thread candies like gumdrops or jellybeans, and make an edible necklace. You could also use marshmallows or dry breakfast cereals, or take a strip of old fabric and tie on some old keys or soda can tabs for a statement piece.

A daughter is a bundle of firsts that excite and delight, giggles that come from deep inside and are always contagious, everything wonderful and precious and your love for her knows no bounds.

——BARBARA CAGE

SHE'LL BE COMIN' 'ROUND THE MOUNTAIN

*She'll be comin' 'round the moun-
tain*

When she comes

(When she comes).

*She'll be comin' 'round the moun-
tain*

When she comes

(When she comes).

*She'll be comin' 'round the moun-
tain,*

*She'll be comin' 'round the moun-
tain,*

*She'll be comin' 'round the moun-
tain*

When she comes

(When she comes).

She'll be drivin' six white horses

When she comes

(When she comes).

She'll be drivin' six white horses

When she comes

(When she comes).

She'll be drivin' six white horses,

She'll be drivin' six white horses,

She'll be drivin' six white horses

When she comes

(When she comes).

Oh, we'll all go out to greet her

When she comes

(When she comes).

Oh, we'll all go out to greet her

When she comes

(When she comes).

Oh, we'll all go out to greet her,

Oh, we'll all go out to greet her,

Oh, we'll all go out to greet her

When she comes

(When she comes).

We will kill the old red rooster

When she comes

(When she comes).

We will kill the old red rooster

When she comes

(When she comes).

We will kill the old red rooster,

We will kill the old red rooster,

We will kill the old red rooster

When she comes

(When she comes).

*Oh, we'll all have chicken and
dumplings*

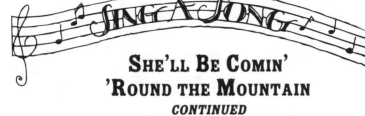

When she comes
(When she comes).
Oh, we'll all have chicken and dumplings
When she comes
(When she comes).
Oh, we'll all have chicken and dumplings,
Oh, we'll all have chicken and dumplings,
Oh, we'll all have chicken and dumplings
When she comes
(When she comes).
She will have to wear pajamas
When she comes
(When she comes).
She will have to wear pajamas
When she comes
(When she comes).
She will have to wear pajamas,

She will have to wear pajamas,
She will have to wear pajamas
When she comes
(When she comes).
She will have to sleep with Grandma
When she comes
(When she comes).
She will have to sleep with Grandma
When she comes
(When she comes).
She will have to sleep with Grandma,
She will have to sleep with Grandma,
She will have to sleep with Grandma
When she comes
(When she comes).

The Story of Goldilocks and the Three Bears

(TRADITIONAL)

 nce upon a time, there was a little girl named Goldilocks. She went for a walk in the forest. Pretty soon, she came upon a house. She knocked and, when no one answered, she walked right in.

At the table in the kitchen, there were three bowls of porridge. Goldilocks was hungry. She tasted the porridge from the first bowl.

"This porridge is too hot!" she exclaimed.

So, she tasted the porridge from the second bowl.

"This porridge is too cold," she said.

So, she tasted the last bowl of porridge.

"Ahhh, this porridge is just right," she said happily and she ate it all up.

After she'd eaten the three bears' breakfasts she decided she was feeling a little tired. So, she walked into the living room where she saw three chairs. Goldilocks sat in the first chair to rest her feet.

"This chair is too big!" she exclaimed.

So she sat in the second chair.

"This chair is too big, too!" she whined.

So she tried the last and smallest chair.

"Ahhh, this chair is just right," she sighed. But just as she settled down into the chair to rest, it broke into pieces!

Goldilocks was very tired by this time, so she went upstairs to the bedroom. She lay down in the first bed, but it was too hard. Then she lay in the second bed, but it was too soft. Then she lay down in the third bed and it was just right. Goldilocks fell asleep. As she was sleeping, the three bears came home.

"Someone's been eating my porridge," growled the Papa bear.

"Someone's been eating my porridge," said the Mama bear.

"Someone's been eating my porridge and they ate it all up!" cried the Baby bear.

"Someone's been sitting in my chair," growled the Papa bear.

"Someone's been sitting in my chair," said the Mama bear.

"Someone's been sitting in my chair and they've broken it all to pieces," cried the Baby bear. They decided to look around some more and when they got upstairs to the bedroom, Papa bear growled, "Someone's been sleeping in my bed."

"Someone's been sleeping in my bed, too," said Mama bear.

"Someone's been sleeping in my bed and she's still there!" exclaimed Baby bear.

Just then, Goldilocks woke up and saw the three bears. She screamed, "Help!" And she jumped up and ran out of the room. Goldilocks ran down the stairs, opened the door, and ran away into the forest. And she never returned to the home of the three bears.

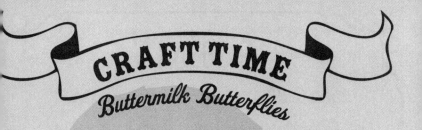

It is important to use full-fat buttermilk in this recipe for best flavor and texture. If you can't get whole buttermilk, use half buttermilk and half sour cream.

Ingredients

YIELDS 60 COOKIES

- 5 cups flour
- 2 cups sugar
- 2 teaspoons baking powder
- 1 teaspoon freshly grated nutmeg
- 1 teaspoon salt
- ½ cup shortening
- 1 cup thick buttermilk
- 3 eggs
- 2 teaspoons vanilla
- 1 teaspoon baking soda

1. Mix flour, sugar, baking powder, nutmeg, and salt. Cut in shortening until mixture looks like coarse crumbs.

2. Mix buttermilk, eggs, vanilla, and baking soda. Stir into flour mixture until it forms a ball. Chill 1 hour, or overnight.

3. Preheat oven to 375°F. Line baking sheets with parchment.

4. Roll dough out on a floured surface to ¼" thick. Cut in butterfly shapes. Sprinkle with sugar; arrange on baking sheets.

5. Bake 15 minutes, or until done. Cool completely.

POEMS

Little Bo Peep

Little Bo Peep has lost her
sheep
And can't tell where to find
them;
Leave them alone, and they'll
come home,
And bring their tails behind
them.

Ring Around the Roses

Ring around the roses,
A pocket full of posies,
Ashes! Ashes!
We all fall down!

Pat-a-Cake

Pat-a-cake, pat-a-cake,
baker's man,
Bake me a cake as
fast as you can.
Roll it, and pat it,
and mark it with a "B"
And put it in the oven
for Baby and me.

Bonny Lass

Bonny lass, pretty lass,
Wilt thou be mine?
Thou shalt not wash dishes
Nor yet serve the swine,
Thou shalt sit on a cushion
And sew a fine seam,
And thou shalt eat strawber-
ries,
Sugar, and cream.

White Butterflies

BY ALGERNON CHARLES SWINBURNE

Fly, white butterflies, out to sea,
Frail, pale wings for the
wind to try,
Small white wings that
we scarce can see,
Fly!
Some fly light as a laugh of glee,
Some fly soft as a long, low
sigh;
All to the haven where each
would be,
Fly!

MOVIES YOUR LITTLE GIRL WILL LOVE!

- *A Little Princess*
- *Pippi Longstocking*
- *Madeline*
- *Harriet the Spy*
- *Heidi*
- *Matilda*
- *Cinderella*
- *The Little Mermaid*
- *Sleeping Beauty*
- *Mary Poppins*
- *The Secret Garden*
- *Alice in Wonderland*
- *Little Women*
- *Tangled*
- *The Wizard of Oz*
- *Mulan*
- *Wild Hearts Can't Be Broken*
- *The Princess Diaries*

SONGS THAT CELEBRATE YOUR DAUGHTER

- "Thank Heaven for Little Girls" by Maurice Chevalier
- "In My Daughter's Eyes" by Martina McBride
- "Butterfly Kisses" by Bob Carlisle
- "Isn't She Lovely" by Stevie Wonder
- "My Little Girl" by Tim McGraw
- "Daughters" by John Mayer
- "The Makings of You" by Curtis Mayfield
- "I Loved Her First" by Heartland
- "Father and Daughter" by Paul Simon
- "Turn Around" by Diana Ross
- "Cinderella" by Steven Curtis Chapman

POEMS

Ladybug, Ladybug Fly Away Home

Ladybug! Ladybug!
Fly away home.
Your house is on fire.
And your children all gone.
All except one,
And that's little Ann,
For she crept under
The frying pan.

Mary, Mary, Quite Contrary

Mary, Mary, quite contrary,
How does your garden grow?
With silver bells, and cockle-
shells,
And pretty maids all in a row.

Sing a Song of Sixpence

Sing a song of sixpence,
A pocket full of rye:
Four and twenty blackbirds
Baked in a pie!
When the pie was opened
The birds began to sing;
Was that not a dainty dish
To set before the king?
The king was in his counting-
house,
Counting out his money;
The queen was in the parlor,
Eating bread and honey.
The maid was in the garden,
Hanging out the clothes;
When down came a blackbird
And snapped off her nose.

There Was an Old Woman

There was an old woman who
lived in a shoe.
She had so many children she
didn't know what to do.
She gave them some broth without any bread.
She whipped them all soundly
and put them to bed.

The Goose-Girl

BY THE BROTHERS GRIMM

he king of a great land died, and left his queen to take care of their only child. This child was a daughter, who was very beautiful; and her mother loved her dearly, and was very kind to her. And there was a good fairy too, who was fond of the princess, and helped her mother to watch over her. When she grew up, she was betrothed to a prince who lived a great way off; and as the time drew near for her to be married, she got ready to set off on her journey to his country. Then the queen her mother packed up a great many costly things; jewels, and gold, and silver; trinkets, fine dresses, and in short everything that became a royal bride. And she gave her a waiting-maid to ride with her, and give her into the bridegroom's hands; and each had a horse for the journey. Now the princess's horse was the fairy's gift, and it was called Falada, and could speak.

When the time came for them to set out, the fairy went into her bed-chamber, and took a little knife, and cut off a lock of her hair, and gave it to the princess, and said, "Take care of it, dear child; for it is a charm that may be of use to you on the road." Then they all took a sorrowful leave of the princess; and she put the lock of hair into her bosom, got upon her horse, and set off on her journey to her bridegroom's kingdom.

One day, as they were riding along by a brook, the princess began to feel very thirsty: and she said to her maid, "Pray get down, and fetch me some water in my golden cup out of yonder brook, for I want to drink." "Nay," said the maid, "if you are thirsty, get off yourself, and stoop down by the water and drink; I shall not be your waiting-maid any longer." Then she was so thirsty that she got down, and knelt over the little brook, and drank; for she was frightened, and dared not bring out her golden cup; and she wept and said, "Alas! what will become of me?" And the lock answered her, and said:

"Alas! alas! if thy mother knew it,

Sadly, sadly, would she rue it."

But the princess was very gentle and meek, so she said nothing to her maid's ill behavior, but got upon her horse again.

Then all rode farther on their journey, till the day grew so warm, and the sun so scorching, that the bride began to feel very thirsty again; and at last, when they came to a river, she forgot her maid's rude speech, and said, "Pray get down, and fetch me some water to drink in my golden cup." But the maid answered her, and even spoke more haughtily than before: "Drink if you will, but I shall not be your waiting-maid." Then the princess was so thirsty that she got off her horse, and lay down, and held her head over the running stream, and cried and said, "What will become of me?" And the lock of hair answered her again:

"Alas! alas! if thy mother knew it,

Sadly, sadly, would she rue it."

And as she leaned down to drink, the lock of hair fell from her bosom, and floated away with the water. Now she was so frightened that she did not see it; but her maid saw it, and was very glad, for she knew the charm; and she saw that the poor bride would be in her power, now that she had lost the hair. So when the bride had done drinking, and would have got upon Falada again, the maid said, "I shall ride upon Falada, and you may have my horse instead"; so she was forced to give up her horse, and soon afterwards to take off her royal clothes and put on her maid's shabby ones.

At last, as they drew near the end of their journey, this treacherous servant threatened to kill her mistress if she ever told anyone what had happened. But Falada saw it all, and marked it well.

Then the waiting-maid got upon Falada, and the real bride rode upon the other horse, and they went on in this way till at last they came to the royal court. There was great joy at their coming, and the prince flew to meet them, and lifted the maid from her horse, thinking she was the one who was to be his wife; and she was led upstairs to the royal chamber; but the true princess was told to stay in the court below.

Now the old king happened just then to have nothing else to do; so he amused himself by sitting at his kitchen window, looking at what was going on; and he saw her in the courtyard. As she looked very pretty, and too delicate for a waiting-maid, he went up into the royal chamber to ask the bride who it was she had brought with her, that was thus left standing in the court below. "I brought her with me for the sake of her company on the road," said she; "pray give the girl some work to do, that she may not be idle." The old king could not for some time think of any work for her to do; but at last he said, "I have a lad who takes care of my geese; she may go and help him." Now the name of this lad, that the real bride was to help in watching the king's geese, was Curdken.

But the false bride said to the prince, "Dear husband, pray do me one piece of kindness." "That I will," said the prince. "Then tell one of your slaughterers to cut off the head of the horse I rode upon, for it was very unruly, and plagued me sadly on the road"; but the truth was, she was very much afraid lest Falada should some day or other speak, and tell all she had done to the princess. She carried her point, and the faithful Falada was killed; but when the true princess heard of it, she wept, and begged the man to nail up Falada's head against a large dark gate of the city, through which she had to pass every morning and evening, that there she might still see him sometimes. Then the slaughterer said he would do as she wished; and cut off the head, and nailed it up under the dark gate.

Early the next morning, as she and Curdken went out through the gate, she said sorrowfully:

"Falada, Falada, there thou hangest!"

and the head answered:

"Bride, bride, there thou gangest!

Alas! alas! if thy mother knew it,

Sadly, sadly, would she rue it."

Then they went out of the city, and drove the geese on. And when she came to the meadow, she sat down upon a bank there, and let down her waving locks of hair, which were all of pure silver; and when Curdken saw it glitter in the sun, he ran up, and would have pulled some of the locks out, but she cried:

"Blow, breezes, blow!

Let Curdken's hat go!

Blow, breezes, blow!

Let him after it go!

O'er hills, dales, and rocks,

Away be it whirl'd

Till the silvery locks

Are all comb'd and curl'd!"

Then there came a wind, so strong that it blew off Curdken's hat; and away it flew over the hills: and he was forced to turn and run after it; till, by the time he came back, she had done combing and curling her hair, and had put it up again safe. Then he was very angry and sulky, and would not speak to her at all; but they watched the geese until it grew dark in the evening, and then drove them homewards.

The next morning, as they were going through the dark gate, the poor girl looked up at Falada's head, and cried:

"Falada, Falada, there thou hangest!"

and the head answered:

"Bride, bride, there thou gangest!

Alas! alas! if thy mother knew it,

Sadly, sadly, would she rue it."

Then she drove on the geese, and sat down again in the meadow, and began to comb out her hair as before; and Curdken ran up to her, and wanted to take hold of it; but she cried out quickly:

"Blow, breezes, blow!

Let Curdken's hat go!

Blow, breezes, blow!

Let him after it go!

O'er hills, dales, and rocks,

Away be it whirl'd

Till the silvery locks

Are all comb'd and curl'd!"

Then the wind came and blew away his hat; and off it flew a great way, over the hills and far away, so that he had to run after it; and when he came back she had bound up her hair again, and all was safe. So they watched the geese till it grew dark.

In the evening, after they came home, Curdken went to the old king, and said, "I cannot have that strange girl to help me to keep the geese any longer." "Why?" said the king. "Because, instead of doing any good, she does nothing but tease me all day long." Then the king made him tell him what had happened. And Curdken said, "When we go in the morning through the dark gate with our flock of geese, she cries and talks with the head of a horse that hangs upon the wall, and says:

'Falada, Falada, there thou hangest!'

and the head answers:

'Bride, bride, there thou gangest!

Alas! alas! if thy mother knew it,

Sadly, sadly, would she rue it.'"

And Curdken went on telling the king what had happened upon the meadow where the geese fed; how his hat was blown away; and how he was forced to run after it, and to leave his flock of geese to themselves. But the old king told the boy to go out again the next day: and when morning came, he placed himself behind the dark gate, and heard how she spoke to Falada, and how Falada answered. Then he went into the field, and hid himself in a bush by the meadow's side; and he soon saw with his own eyes how they drove the flock of geese; and how, after a little time, she let down her hair that glittered in the sun. And then he heard her say:

"Blow, breezes, blow!
Let Curdken's hat go!
Blow, breezes, blow!
Let him after it go!
O'er hills, dales, and rocks,
Away be it whirl'd
Till the silvery locks
Are all comb'd and curl'd!"

And soon came a gale of wind, and carried away Curdken's hat, and away went Curdken after it, while the girl went on combing and curling her hair. All this the old king saw: so he went home without being seen; and when the little goose-girl came back in the evening he called her aside, and asked her why she did so: but she burst into tears, and said, "That I must not tell you or any man, or I shall lose my life."

But the old king begged so hard, that she had no peace till she had told him all the tale, from beginning to end, word for word. And it was very lucky for her that she did so, for when she had done the king ordered royal clothes to be put upon her, and gazed on her with wonder, she was so beautiful. Then he called his son and told him that he had only a false bride; for that she was merely a waiting-maid, while the true bride stood by. And the young king rejoiced when he saw her beauty, and heard how meek and patient she had been; and without saying anything to the false bride, the king ordered a great feast to be got ready for all his court. The bridegroom sat at the top, with the false princess on one side, and the true one on the other; but nobody knew her again, for her beauty was quite dazzling to their eyes; and she did not seem at all like the little goosegirl, now that she had her brilliant dress on.

When they had eaten and drank, and were very merry, the old king said he would tell them a tale. So he began, and told all the story of the princess, as if it was one that he had once heard; and he asked the true waiting-maid what she thought ought to be done to anyone who would behave thus. "Nothing better," said this false bride, "than that she should be thrown into a cask stuck round with sharp nails, and that two white horses should be put to it, and should drag it from street to street till she was dead." "Thou art she!" said the old king; "and as thou has judged thyself, so shall it be done to thee." And the young king was then married to his true wife, and they reigned over the kingdom in peace and happiness all their lives; and the good fairy came to see them, and restored the faithful Falada to life again.

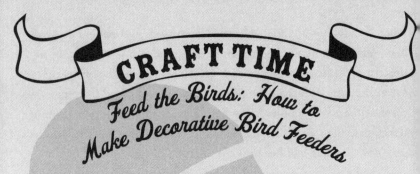

CRAFT TIME

Feed the Birds: How to Make Decorative Bird Feeders

Get in touch with nature and wildlife with the creation of your very own handmade birdfeeder. Your daughter will be as delighted to make it as the birds will be to eat it!

What You'll Need:

- An egg white
- Birdseed of any variety
- Cookie cutter(s)
- A few slices of bread, old or new
- A straw
- A pastry brush
- Pieces of ribbon, yarn, or twine

1. Preheat the oven to 350°F. Beat the egg white until frothy in a small bowl, and pour the birdseed in a shallow dish.

2. Use the cookie cutters to make shapes in the slices of bread. With the straw, punch out a hole for the string about a quarter of an inch from the edge.

3. Brush the cut outs with the egg whites, and then press them into the birdseed. Bake for about 10 minutes.

4. When cooled, thread the string through the hole and hang in a spot where you can watch the birds enjoy!

A daughter may outgrow your lap, but she will never outgrow your heart.

—UNKNOWN

POEMS

Old Mother Hubbard

Old Mother Hubbard
Went to the cupboard
To give the poor dog a bone:
When she came there
The cupboard was bare,
And so the poor dog had none.
She went to the baker's
To buy him some bread;
When she came back
The dog was dead!
She went to the undertaker's
To buy him a coffin;
When she came back
The dog was laughing.
She took a clean dish
to get him some tripe;
When she came back
He was smoking his pipe.
She went to the alehouse
To get him some beer;
When she came back
The dog sat in a chair.
She went to the tavern
For white wine and red;
When she came back

The dog stood on his head.
She went to the fruiterer's
To buy him some fruit;
When she came back
He was playing the flute.
She went to the tailor's
To buy him a coat;
When she came back
He was riding a goat.
She went to the hatter's
To buy him a hat;
When she came back
He was feeding her cat.
She went to the barber's
To buy him a wig,
When she came back
He was dancing a jig.
She went to the cobbler's
To buy him some shoes;
When she came back
He was reading the news.
She went to the seamstress
To buy him some linen;
When she came back
The dog was spinning.
She went to the hosier's
To buy him some hose;

POEMS

When she came back
He was dressed in his clothes.
The Dame made a curtsy,
The dog made a bow;
The Dame said, Your servant;
The dog said, Bow-wow.
This wonderful dog
Was Dame Hubbard's delight,
He could read, he could dance,
He could sing, he could write;
She gave him rich dainties
Whenever he fed,
And erected this monument
When he was dead.

What Does Little Birdie Say?

BY ALFRED, LORD TENNYSON

What does little birdie say
In her nest at peep of day?
Let me fly, says little birdie,
Mother, let me fly away.
Birdie, rest a little longer,
Till thy little wings are stronger.
So she rests a little longer,
Then she flies away.

What does little baby say,
In her bed at peep of day.
Baby says, like little birdie,
Let me rise and fly away.
Baby, sleep a little longer,
Till thy little limbs are stronger.
If she sleeps a little longer,
Baby too shall fly away.

Little Miss Muffet

Little Miss Muffet,
Sat on a tuffet,
Eating some curds and whey;
There came a spider,
And sat down beside her,
And frightened Miss
Muffet away.

Little Girl

Little girl, little girl, where
have you been?
Gathering roses to give
to the Queen.
Little girl, little girl, what
gave she you?
She gave me a diamond as
big as my shoe.

The Real Princess
(The Princess and the Pea)

BY HANS CHRISTIAN ANDERSEN

here was once a prince who wanted to marry a princess. But she must be a real princess, mind you. So he traveled all round the world, seeking such a one, but everywhere something was in the way. Not that there was any lack of princesses, but he could not seem to make out whether they were real princesses; there was always something not quite satisfactory. Therefore, home he came again, quite out of spirits, for he wished so much to marry a real princess.

One evening a terrible storm came on. It thundered and lightened, and the rain poured down; indeed, it was quite fearful. In the midst of it there came a knock at the town gate, and the old king went out to open it.

It was a princess who stood outside. But O dear, what a state she was in from the rain and bad weather! The water dropped from her hair and clothes, it ran in at the tips of her shoes and out at the heels; yet she insisted she was a real princess.

"Very well," thought the old queen; "that we shall presently see." She said nothing, but went into the bedchamber and took off all the bedding, then laid a pea on the sacking of the bedstead. Having done this, she took twenty mattresses and laid them upon the pea and placed twenty eider-down beds on top of the mattresses.

The princess lay upon this bed all the night. In the morning she was asked how she had slept.

"Oh, most miserably!" she said. "I scarcely closed my eyes the whole night through. I cannot think what there could have been in the bed. I lay upon something so hard that I am quite black and blue all over. It is dreadful!"

It was now quite evident that she was a real princess, since through twenty mattresses and twenty eider-down beds she had felt the pea. None but a real princess could have such delicate feeling.

So the prince took her for his wife, for he knew that in her he had found a true princess. And the pea was preserved in the cabinet of curiosities, where it is still to be seen unless some one has stolen it.

And this, mind you, is a real story.

Traditional Games for Girls

he games below have been favorites of little girls for centuries. Share your fond memories with your daughter and teach her how to play these classics!

HOPSCOTCH
Before you begin:
Decide where you'd like to play. You can use sidewalk chalk on asphalt outside, or use masking tape to create a design inside. Make sure the squares are large enough to fit your foot!

Design your hopscotch squares as creatively as you'd like and number them, starting with 1. Then find a small object or marker to throw. Outside, a small stone is fitting, and inside, you could use a beanbag, a button, or any other small object.

The goal:
To complete the course, landing your marker on each square in order, without losing a turn. The first person to land their marker on each number and complete the course wins the game!

To play:
The object of the game is to throw your marker so it lands inside each square without bouncing out or touching the border. If your marker does not land inside the border, your turn is over and play passes to the next person. If it does land inside, hop on one foot through the hopscotch squares in order (unless you reach two squares side by side, in which case you can use both feet, one for each square), hopping *over* the square with your marker in it. If you hop on or outside the lines or hop in a square out of order, your turn is over.

At the last square in your course, turn around on one foot and make your way back through the board. When you come to your marker, stay on one foot, pick it up, and skip over the square it was in until you reach the beginning again.

If you reach the beginning without a misstep, then pass the marker on to the next person.

MOTHER MAY I

Before you begin:

You'll need at least three players.

Choose one player to be "Mother" (or "Father").

To play:

Line up your players, or "children," facing "Mother" about ten or so feet away, or on the opposite sides of a room.

The players, one by one, ask Mother if they can move forward a certain number of steps (for example, "Mother, may I take five steps forward?"). They can also fill in the blank with different requests, like:

- "Mother, may I take (#) steps forward?"
- "Mother, may I take (#) giant steps forward?"
- "Mother, may I take (#) baby steps forward?"

Mother is allowed to respond however she pleases and players must follow the Mother's instructions. If she agrees to the request, she will answer "Yes, _____, you may take one step forward." She may also make another suggestion, answering "No, you may not, but you can _____ instead."

Mother doesn't want the children to reach her too quickly, so she may decide to:

- Reduce the original child's request, allowing a smaller number of steps, for example.

- Tell a player to take (#) steps backward, run backward for (#) seconds, walk backward until she says "stop," or even tell the player to go back to the starting line.

The children must obey Mother or they're out of the game.

The first of the children to reach Mother wins the game. The winner then becomes the next Mother or Father and a new game begins!

DOUBLE DUTCH

Before you begin:

You'll need two jump ropes, and at least three people: two turners to swing the ropes, and at least one jumper!

To play:

First, the turners take the ropes, one in each hand, and hold their hands at waist height, shoulder width apart. They begin swinging the jump ropes simultaneously in opposite directions, their left arms swinging the rope clockwise, their rights arms turning the other rope counterclockwise, making large arcs with the ropes. When the left hand is up, the right hand should be down. For spinners rhythm is important, along with deciding how fast or as slow they'd like to turn the ropes.

The jumper then jumps into the ropes when the rope closest to them hits the ground, jumping in at a diagonal angle. (You can start in the middle of the ropes before they start being turned if you find it too difficult to jump in while the ropes are swinging.) For the jumper, timing and coordination are essential to learning to jump Double Dutch.

The jumper(s) need to move their feet alternately to jump over the ropes as they pass by. You can play to see how many jumps you can do in a certain time, experiment with different freestyle tricks, or jump along to schoolyard Double Dutch rhymes and verses!

HOPSCOTCH/JUMP ROPE RHYMES

Fudge, fudge, call the judge,
Mama's got a new-born baby
It's not a boy
It's not a girl
It's just an ordinary baby
Wrap it up in tissue paper,
Send it down the elevator.
First floor—Miss!
Second floor—Miss! (continue counting until jumper misses)

Cinderella, dressed in yellow
Went upstairs to kiss a fellow
Made a mistake
Kissed a snake
How many doctors
Did it take?
1, 2, 3, 4 (continue counting until the jumper misses)

One, two, buckle my shoe
Three, four, close the door
Five, six, pick up sticks
Seven, eight, shut the gate
Nine, ten, start again.

Charlie Chaplin went to France
To teach the ladies how to dance.
First the heel, then the toe,
Then the splits, and around you go!

Call for the doctor, call for the nurse,
And call for the lady with the alligator purse!
In came the doctor, in came the nurse,
And in came the lady with the alligator purse.
Out went the doctor, out went the nurse,
And out went the lady with the alligator purse!

Not last night but the night before
Forty-four robbers came knocking at my door!
As I ran out, they ran in,
Asked them what they wanted, and they said:
Spanish dancer, turn around (turn while jumping)
Spanish dancer, touch the ground (bend to touch the ground)
Spanish dancer, do a high kick (kick)
Spanish dancer, get out of town quick! (jump out of the ropes)

All in together, birds of a feather:
January, February, March, April, May, etc. (each player jumps in during the month they were born)

Ice cream soda, Delaware Punch,
Tell me the name of my honey-bunch.
A, B, C (continue until the jumper misses)

I'm a little Dutch girl
Dressed in blue,
Here are the things
I like to do:
Salute to the captain (salute)
Bow to the queen (bow)
Turn my back on the submarine (turn around and face the other direction)
I can do the tap dance (dance)
I can do the splits (jump up high with legs apart)
I can do the hokey pokey (turn yourself around)
Just like this!

Miss Mary Mack, Mack, Mack,
All dressed in black, black, black,
With silver buttons, buttons, buttons,
All down her back, back, back,
She asked her mother, mother, mother,
For fifty cents, cents, cents,

To see the elephants, elephants, elephants,
Jump the fence, fence, fence,
They jumped so high, high, high,
They touched the sky, sky, sky,
And didn't come back, back, back,
Till the fourth of July, ly, ly.

Ice cream, soda pop, cherry on top,
Who's your best friend?
I forgot!
A, B, C (continue until the jumper misses)

Briar Rose
(Sleeping Beauty)

BY THE BROTHERS GRIMM

 king and queen once upon a time reigned in a country a great way off, where there were in those days fairies. Now this king and queen had plenty of money, and plenty of fine clothes to wear, and plenty of good things to eat and drink, and a coach to ride out in every day: but though they had been married many years they had no children, and this grieved them very much indeed. But one day as the queen was walking by the side of the river, at the bottom of the garden, she saw a poor little fish, that had thrown itself out of the water, and lay gasping and nearly dead on the bank. Then the queen took pity on the little fish, and threw it back again into the river; and before it swam away it lifted its head out of the water and said, "I know what your wish is, and it shall be fulfilled, in return for your kindness to me—you will soon have a daughter."

What the little fish had foretold soon came to pass; and the queen had a little girl, so very beautiful that the king could not cease looking on it for joy, and said he would hold a great feast and make merry, and show the child to all the land. So he asked his kinsmen, and nobles, and friends, and neighbors. But the queen said, "I will have the fairies also, that they might be kind and good to our little daughter." Now there were thirteen fairies in the kingdom; but as the king and queen had only twelve golden dishes for them to eat out of, they were forced to leave one of the fairies without asking her. So twelve fairies came, each with a high red cap on her head, and red shoes with high heels on her feet, and a long white wand in her hand: and after the feast was over they gathered round in a ring and gave all their best gifts to the little princess. One gave her goodness, another beauty, another riches, and so on till she had all that was good in the world.

Just as eleven of them had done blessing her, a great noise was heard in the courtyard, and word was brought that the thirteenth fairy was come, with a black cap on her head, and black shoes on her feet, and a broomstick in her hand: and presently up she came into the dining-hall. Now, as she had not been asked to the feast she was very angry, and scolded the king and queen very much, and set to work to take her revenge. So she cried out, "The king's daughter shall, in her fifteenth year, be wounded by a spindle, and fall down dead." Then the twelfth of the friendly fairies, who had not yet given her gift, came forward, and said that the evil wish must be fulfilled, but that she could soften its mischief; so her gift was that the king's daughter, when the spindle wounded her, should not really die, but should only fall asleep for a hundred years.

However, the king hoped still to save his dear child altogether from the threatened evil; so he ordered that all the spindles in the kingdom should be bought up and burnt. But all the gifts of the first eleven fairies were in the meantime fulfilled; for the princess was so beautiful, and well behaved, and good, and wise, that everyone who knew her loved her.

It happened that, on the very day she was fifteen years old, the king and queen were not at home, and she was left alone in the palace. So she roved about by herself, and looked at all the rooms and chambers, till at last she came to an old tower, to which there was a narrow staircase ending with a little door. In the door there was a golden key, and when she turned it the door sprang open, and there sat an old lady spinning away very busily. "Why, how now, good mother," said the princess; "what are you doing there?" "Spinning," said the old lady, and nodded her head, humming a tune, while buzz! went the wheel. "How prettily that little thing turns round!" said the princess, and took the spindle and began to try and spin. But scarcely had she touched it, before the fairy's prophecy was fulfilled; the spindle wounded her, and she fell down lifeless on the ground.

However, she was not dead, but had only fallen into a deep sleep; and the king and the queen, who had just come home, and all their court, fell asleep too; and the horses slept in the stables, and the dogs in the court, the pigeons on the house-top, and the very flies slept upon the walls. Even the fire on the hearth left off blazing, and went to sleep; the jack stopped, and the spit that was turning about with a goose upon it for the king's dinner stood still; and the cook, who was at that moment pulling the kitchen-boy by the hair to give him a box on the ear for something he had done amiss, let him go, and both fell asleep; the butler, who was slyly tasting the ale, fell asleep with the jug at his lips: and thus everything stood still, and slept soundly.

A large hedge of thorns soon grew round the palace, and every year it became higher and thicker; till at last the old palace was surrounded and hidden, so that not even the roof or the chimneys could be seen. But there went a report through all the land of the beautiful sleeping Briar Rose (for so the king's daughter was called): so that, from time to time, several kings' sons came, and tried to break through the thicket into the palace. This, however, none of them could ever do; for the thorns and bushes laid hold of them, as if they were with hands; and there they stuck fast, and died wretchedly.

After many, many years there came a king's son into that land: and an old man told him the story of the thicket of thorns; and how a beautiful palace stood behind it, and how a wonderful princess, called Briar Rose, lay in it asleep, with all her court. He told, too, how he had heard from his grandfather that many, many princes had come, and had tried to break through the thicket, but that they had all stuck fast in it, and died. Then the young prince said, "All this shall not frighten me; I will go and see this Briar Rose." The old man tried to hinder him, but he was bent upon going.

Now that very day the hundred years were ended; and as the prince came to the thicket he saw nothing but beautiful flowering shrubs, through which he went with ease, and they shut in after him as thick as ever. Then he came at last to the palace, and there in the court lay the dogs asleep; and the horses were standing in the stables; and on the roof sat the pigeons fast asleep, with their heads under their wings. And when he came into the palace, the flies were sleeping on the walls; the spit was standing still; the butler had the jug of ale at his lips, going to drink a draught; the maid sat with a fowl in her lap ready to be plucked; and the cook in the kitchen was still holding up her hand, as if she was going to beat the boy.

Then he went on still farther, and all was so still that he could hear every breath he drew; till at last he came to the old tower, and opened the door of the little room in which Briar Rose was; and there she lay, fast asleep on a couch by the window. She looked so beautiful that he could not take his eyes off her, so he stooped down and gave her a kiss. But the moment he kissed her she opened her eyes and awoke, and smiled upon him; and they went out together; and soon the king and queen also awoke, and all the court, and gazed on each other with great wonder. And the horses shook themselves, and the dogs jumped up and barked; the pigeons took their heads from under their wings, and looked about and flew into the fields; the flies on the walls buzzed again; the fire in the kitchen blazed up; round went the jack, and round went the spit, with the goose for the king's dinner upon it; the butler finished his draught of ale; the maid went on plucking the fowl; and the cook gave the boy the box on his ear.

And then the prince and Briar Rose were married, and the wedding feast was given; and they lived happily together all their lives long.

POEMS

The Three Little Kittens

Three little kittens, they
lost their mittens,
And they began to cry,
Oh, mother dear, we sadly fear
That we have lost our mittens.
What! Lost your mittens, you
naughty kittens!
Then you shall have no pie.
Mee-ow, mee-ow, mee-ow,
mee-ow.
You shall have no pie.
The three little kittens, they
found their mittens,
And they began to cry,
Oh, mother dear, see here,
see here,
Our mittens we have found.
Put on your mittens, you
silly kittens,
And you shall have some pie.
Purr-r, purr-r, purr-r,
Oh, let us have some pie.
The three little kittens, they put
on their mittens,
And soon ate up the pie;
Oh, mother dear, we greatly fear
That we have soiled our mittens.

What! Soiled your mittens, you
naughty kittens!
Then they began to sigh,
Mee-ow, mee-ow, mee-ow,
mee-ow.
They began to sigh.
The three little kittens, they
washed their mittens,
And hung them out to dry;
Oh! mother dear, do you not hear
That we have washed our mit-
tens?
What! Washed your mittens,
then you're such good kittens.
But I smell a rat close by
Mee-ow, mee-ow, mee-ow,
mee-ow.
We smell a rat close by.

There Was a Little Girl

BY Henry Wadsworth
Longfellow

There was a little girl
Who had a little curl
Right in the middle of her
forehead.
When she was good
She was very good indeed,
But when she was bad she
was horrid.

Girls are giggles with freckles all over them.

——UNKNOWN

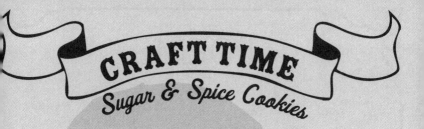

CRAFT TIME
Sugar & Spice Cookies

YIELDS FIVE DOZEN SPICE COOKIES

- 2½ cups all-purpose flour, sifted or stirred before measuring
- ⅛ teaspoon salt
- ½ teaspoon cream of tartar
- ½ teaspoon baking soda
- ½ teaspoon nutmeg
- ¼ teaspoon cinnamon
- ¼ cup shortening
- ¼ cup butter
- 1 cup granulated sugar
- 1 egg
- ⅓ cup milk
- 1 egg white, slightly beaten
- Granulated sugar

1. Sift together the flour, salt, cream of tartar, baking soda, nutmeg, and cinnamon.

2. In a separate mixing bowl, cream together the shortening and butter with sugar until well mixed and fluffy; carefully add in the egg and milk. When well mixed, slowly add in flour mixture. Chill the dough for two to three hours.

3. When dough has chilled, dust the countertop with flour and roll the dough out to about ¼-inch thickness; cut out with cookie cutters. Place cookies on cookie sheet and brush the top with the egg white. Sprinkle with sugar and bake at 375°F for about ten minutes or until edges are golden.

POEMS

Good Night and Good Morning

BY RICHARD
MONCKTON MILNES,
LORD HOUGHTON

A fair little girl sat under a tree,

Sewing as long as her
eyes could see;

Then smoothed her work, and
folded it right,

And said, "Dear work, good
night! good night!"

Such a number of rooks came
over her head,

Crying, "Caw! Caw!" on
their way to bed;

She said, as she watched their
curious flight,

"Little black things, good night!
good night!"

The horses neighed, and the
oxen lowed,

The sheep's "Bleat! bleat!"
came over the road;

All seeming to say, with a quiet
delight,

"Good little girl, good night!
good night!"

She did not say to the sun,
"Good night!"

Though she saw him there
like a ball of light,

For she knew he had God's
time to keep

All over the world, and
never could sleep.

The tall pink foxglove
bowed his head,

The violets curtsied and
went to bed;

And good little Lucy
tied up her hair,

And said on her knees
her favorite prayer.

And while on her
pillow she softly lay,

She knew nothing more
till again it was day;

And all things said to the
beautiful sun,

"Good morning! good morning!
our work is begun!"

WHAT'S IN A NAME?

These lists of popular names in decades past provide a unique opportunity to talk about history and tradition with your daughter. Take time to look back in your family tree and see what names you find!

1920s
- Mary
- Dorothy
- Helen
- Betty
- Margaret
- Ruth
- Virginia
- Doris
- Mildred
- Frances

1930s
- Mary
- Betty
- Barbara
- Shirley
- Patricia
- Dorothy
- Joan
- Margaret
- Nancy
- Helen

1940s
- Mary
- Linda
- Barbara
- Patricia
- Carol
- Sandra
- Nancy
- Sharon
- Judith
- Susan

1950s
- Mary
- Linda
- Patricia
- Susan
- Deborah
- Barbara
- Debra
- Karen
- Nancy
- Donna

1960s
- Lisa
- Mary
- Susan
- Karen
- Kimberly
- Patricia
- Linda
- Donna
- Michelle
- Cynthia

1970s
- Jennifer
- Amy
- Melissa
- Michelle
- Kimberly
- Lisa
- Angela
- Heather
- Stephanie
- Nicole

1980s
- Jessica
- Jennifer
- Amanda
- Ashley
- Sarah
- Stephanie
- Melissa
- Nicole
- Elizabeth
- Heather

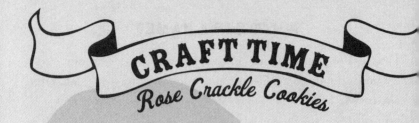

CRAFT TIME
Rose Crackle Cookies

Rose water is an old-fashioned flavor that is regaining popularity. It is sweetly floral and very delicate. For an extra flourish, roll these cookies in pink sugar crystals.

Ingredients

YIELDS 60 COOKIES

- 1 cup unsalted butter
- 2 cups sugar
- 2 eggs
- ½ teaspoon vanilla
- 1 teaspoon rose water
- 2⅔ cups flour
- 1 teaspoon cream of tartar
- 1 teaspoon baking soda
- ½ teaspoon salt
- Sugar with a few drops of rose water in it for rolling

1. Cream butter and 2 cups of sugar until light and fluffy. Add eggs one at a time, beating well after each addition. Add vanilla and rose water; beat until smooth.

2. Blend dry ingredients; stir into butter mixture. Chill 2 hours.

3. Preheat oven to 350°F.

4. Roll tablespoons of cold dough into balls; roll in sugar. Place 2" apart on ungreased baking sheets.

5. Bake 20 minutes. Cool completely.

POEMS

A Game of Fives
BY LEWIS CARROLL

Five little girls, of Five, Four,
Three, Two, One:

Rolling on the hearthrug,
full of tricks and fun.

Five rosy girls, in years from
Ten to Six:

Sitting down to lessons -
no more time for tricks.

Five growing girls, from
Fifteen to Eleven:

Music, Drawing, Languages,
and food enough for seven!

Five winsome girls, from
Twenty to Sixteen:

Each young man that calls, I
say "Now tell me which you
MEAN!"

Five dashing girls, the youngest
Twenty-one:

But, if nobody proposes, what
is there to be done?

Five showy girls - but
Thirty is an age

When girls may be ENGAG-
ING,

but they somehow don't
ENGAGE.

Five dressy girls, of
Thirty-one or more:

So gracious to the shy young
men they snubbed so much
before!

What is Pink?
BY CHRISTINA ROSSETTI

What is pink? A rose is pink
By the fountain's brink.

What is red? A poppy's red
In its barley bed.

What is blue? The sky is blue
Where the clouds float thro'.

What is white? A swan is white
Sailing in the light.

What is yellow? Pears are yellow,

Rich and ripe and mellow.

What is green? The grass is
green

With small flowers between.

What is violet? Clouds are
violet

In the summer twilight,

What is orange? Why, an
orange,

Just an orange!

Rapunzel

BY THE BROTHERS GRIMM

here were once a man and a woman who had long in vain wished for a child. At length the woman hoped that God was about to grant her desire. These people had a little window at the back of their house from which a splendid garden could be seen, which was full of the most beautiful flowers and herbs. It was, however, surrounded by a high wall, and no one dared to go into it because it belonged to an enchantress, who had great power and was dreaded by all the world.

One day the woman was standing by this window and looking down into the garden, when she saw a bed which was planted with the most beautiful rampion (rapunzel), and it looked so fresh and green that she longed for it, she quite pined away, and began to look pale and miserable. Then her husband was alarmed, and asked: "What ails you, dear wife?" "Ah," she replied, "if I can't eat some of the rampion, which is in the garden behind our house, I shall die." The man, who loved her, thought: "Sooner than let your wife die, bring her some of the rampion yourself, let it cost what it will." At twilight, he clambered down over the wall into the garden of the enchantress, hastily clutched a handful of rampion, and took it to his wife. She at once made herself a salad of it, and ate it greedily. It tasted so good to her—so very good, that the next day she longed for it three times as much as before. If he was to have any rest, her husband must once more descend into the garden.

In the gloom of evening therefore, he let himself down again; but when he had clambered down the wall he was terribly afraid, for he saw the enchantress standing before him. "How can you dare," said she with angry look, "descend into my garden and steal my rampion like a thief? You shall suffer for it!" "Ah," answered he, "let mercy take the place of justice, I only made up my mind to do it out of necessity. My wife saw your rampion from the window, and felt such a longing for it that she would have died if she had not got some to eat." Then the enchantress allowed her anger to be softened, and said to him: "If the case be as you say, I will allow you to take away with you as much rampion as you will, only I make one condition, you must give me the child which your wife will bring into the world; it shall be well treated, and I will care for it like a mother." The man in his terror consented to everything, and when the woman was brought to bed, the enchantress appeared at once, gave the child the name of Rapunzel, and took it away with her.

Rapunzel grew into the most beautiful child under the sun. When she was twelve years old, the enchantress shut her into a tower, which lay in a forest, and had neither stairs nor door, but quite at the top was a little window. When the enchantress wanted to go in, she placed herself beneath it and cried:

"Rapunzel, Rapunzel,

Let down your hair to me."

Rapunzel had magnificent long hair, fine as spun gold, and when she heard the voice of the enchantress she unfastened her braided tresses, wound them round one of the hooks of the window above, and then the hair fell twenty ells down, and the enchantress climbed up by it.

After a year or two, it came to pass that the king's son rode through the forest and passed by the tower. Then he heard a song, which was so charming that he stood still and listened. This was Rapunzel, who in her solitude passed her time in letting her sweet voice resound. The king's son wanted to climb up to her, and looked for the door of the tower, but none was to be found. He rode home, but the singing had so deeply touched his heart, that every day he went out into the forest and listened to it. Once when he was thus standing behind a tree, he saw that an enchantress came there, and he heard how she cried:

"Rapunzel, Rapunzel,

Let down your hair to me."

Then Rapunzel let down the braids of her hair, and the enchantress climbed up to her. "If that is the ladder by which one mounts, I too will try my fortune," said he, and the next day when it began to grow dark, he went to the tower and cried:

"Rapunzel, Rapunzel,

Let down your hair to me."

Immediately the hair fell down and the king's son climbed up.

At first Rapunzel was terribly frightened when a man, such as her eyes had never yet beheld, came to her; but the king's son began to talk to her quite like a friend, and told her that his heart had been so stirred that it had let him have no rest, and he had been forced to see her. Then Rapunzel lost her fear, and when he asked her if she would take him for her husband, and she saw that he was young and handsome, she thought: "He will love me more than old Dame Gothel does"; and she said yes, and laid her hand in his. She said: "I will willingly go away with you, but I do not know how to get down. Bring with you a skein of silk every time that you come, and I will weave a ladder with it, and when that is ready I will descend, and you will take me on your horse." They agreed that until that time he should come to her every evening, for the old woman came by day.

The enchantress remarked nothing of this, until once Rapunzel said to her: "Tell me, Dame Gothel, how it happens that you are so much heavier for me to draw up than the young king's son — he is with me in a moment." "Ah! you wicked child," cried the enchantress. "What do I hear you say! I thought I had separated you from all the world, and yet you have deceived me!" In her anger she clutched Rapunzel's beautiful tresses, wrapped them twice round her left hand, seized a pair of scissors with the right, and snip, snap, they were cut off, and the lovely braids lay on the ground. And she was so pitiless that she took poor Rapunzel into a desert where she had to live in great grief and misery.

On the same day that she cast out Rapunzel, however, the enchantress fastened the braids of hair, which she had cut off, to the hook of the window, and when the king's son came and cried:

"Rapunzel, Rapunzel,

Let down your hair to me."

she let the hair down. The king's son ascended, but instead of finding his dearest Rapunzel, he found the enchantress, who gazed at him with wicked and venomous looks. "Aha!" she cried mockingly, "you would fetch your dearest, but the beautiful bird sits no longer singing in the nest; the cat has got it, and will scratch out your eyes as well. Rapunzel is lost to you; you will never see her again."

The king's son was beside himself with pain, and in his despair he leapt down from the tower. He escaped with his life, but the thorns into which he fell pierced his eyes. Then he wandered quite blind about the forest, ate nothing but roots and berries, and did naught but lament and weep over the loss of his dearest wife. Thus he roamed about in misery for some years, and at length came to the desert where Rapunzel, with the twins to which she had given birth, a boy and a girl, lived in wretchedness. He heard a voice, and it seemed so familiar to him that he went towards it, and when he approached, Rapunzel knew him and fell on his neck and wept. Two of her tears wetted his eyes and they grew clear again, and he could see with them as before. He led her to his kingdom where he was joyfully received, and they lived for a long time afterwards, happy and contented.

Little girls dance their way into your heart, whirling on the tips of angel wings, scattering gold dust and kisses in our paths.

—Unknown

BEDTIME PRAYERS

Grace

Thank you for the world so sweet,
Thank you for the food we eat.
Thank you for the birds that sing,
Thank you, God, for everything.
— E. Rutter Leatham

Now I Lay Me Down

Now I lay me down to sleep,
I pray the Lord my soul to keep,
Lord, be with me through the
night
And keep me 'til the
morning light.

A Child's Evening Hymn

I hear no voice, I feel no touch,
I see no glory bright;
But yet I know that God is near,
In darkness as in light.
God watches ever by my side,
And hears my whispered
prayer:
A God of love for a little child
Both night and day does care.

Angel Blessing at Bedtime

Angels bless and angels keep
Angels guard me while I sleep
Bless my heart and bless
my home
Bless my spirit as I roam
Guide and guard me through
the night
And wake me with the morn-
ing's light.
Amen

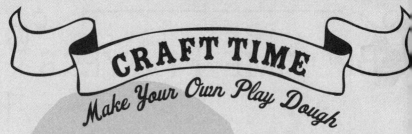

CRAFT TIME
Make Your Own Play Dough

Making play dough is a simple and fun activity to try with your little girl. She can help with the recipe *and* enjoy hours of fun shaping and molding her very own play dough! Don't forget to store your play dough in an air-tight container when you're done having fun!

What You'll Need:

- ➼ 2 cups flour
- ➼ 2 cups warm water
- ➼ 1 cup salt
- ➼ 2 tablespoons vegetable oil
- ➼ 1 tablespoon cream of tartar
- ➼ Food coloring gel (if desired)

1. Mix all of the ingredients (except for the food coloring) together in a pot on the stove over low heat.

2. As you stir, the dough will thicken and then pull away from the sides to the center.

3. Continue to stir and cook until the dough is no longer sticky, but has dry, dough-like texture.

4. Remove the dough so it can cool, and then knead the dough until there are no more lumps.

5. Now you are ready to color the play dough, if you'd like. Separate the dough into pieces and roll the pieces into balls. Then poke a hole into the center and use this hole to put a few drops of dye in. (This way the food coloring won't come into direct contact with your skin until you've worked it into the dough. You could use plastic wrap or gloves to work the food coloring through as well.) Knead the dough to distribute the dye, adding more food coloring until the desired color is reached.

BOOKS TO READ TO YOUR DAUGHTER

Mystery, danger, love, excitement, fantasy! Here are some tales of faraway lands and places that can only be reached when you open a book and read with your daughter. Let your imaginations run wild together as you explore the worlds and unravel the stories beloved by girls for centuries.

- *Pat the Bunny*
  by Dorothy Kunhardt

- *Goodnight Moon*
  by Margaret Wise Brown

- *Madeline*
  by Ludwig Bemelmans

- *Eloise*
  by Kay Thompson

- *Make Way for Ducklings*
  by Robert McCloskey

- *Corduroy*
  by Don Freeman

- *Olivia*
  by Ian Falconer

- *Are You My Mother?*
  by P.D. Eastman

- *The Velveteen Rabbit*
  by Margery Williams

- *Junie B. Jones* series
  by Barbara Park

- *Amelia Bedelia* series
  by Peggy Parish

- *Sarah, Plain and Tall*
  Patricia MacLachlan

- *Alice's Adventures in Wonderland*
  by Lewis Carroll

- *Anne of Green Gables*
  by Lucy Maud Montgomery

- *A Little Princess*
  by Frances Hodgson Burnett

- *The Secret Garden*
  by Frances Hodgson Burnett

- *Matilda*
  by Roald Dahl

- *Ramona*
  by Beverly Cleary

LULLABIES

Hush, Little Baby

Hush, little baby, don't
say a word.

Papa's gonna buy you
a mockingbird

And if that mockingbird won't
sing,

Papa's gonna buy you a
diamond ring

And if that diamond
ring turns brass,

Papa's gonna buy you
a looking glass

And if that looking
glass gets broke,

Papa's gonna buy you a billy
goat

And if that billy goat won't pull,

Papa's gonna buy you a cart
and bull

And if that cart and bull turn
over,

Papa's gonna buy you a dog
named Rover

And if that dog named Rover
won't bark

Papa's gonna buy you a
horse and cart

And if that horse and cart
fall down,

You'll still be the sweetest little
baby in town.

All the Pretty Horses

Hush-a-bye, don't you cry,

Go to sleep my little baby.

When you wake you shall have

All the pretty little horses.

Black and bays, dapples and
grays,

All the pretty little horses.

Hush-a-bye, don't you cry,

Go to sleep my little baby.

Hush-a-bye, don't you cry,

Go to sleep my little baby.

When you wake you shall have

All the pretty little horses.

Lullabies

Hush-a-Bye Baby

Hush-a-bye, Baby, upon
the tree top,

When the wind blows the
cradle will rock;

When the bough breaks the
cradle will fall,

Down tumbles cradle, Baby,
and all.

Brahms's Lullaby (Lullaby and Goodnight)

Lullaby and goodnight, with
roses bedight

With lilies o'er spread is
baby's wee bed

Lay thee down now and rest,
may thy slumber be blessed

Lay thee down now and rest,
may thy slumber be blessed

Lullaby and goodnight, thy
mother's delight

Bright angels beside my
darling abide

They will guard thee at rest,
thou shalt wake on my breast

They will guard thee at rest,
thou shalt wake on my breast

Gaelic Lullaby (traditional)

Hush, the waves are rolling in,

White with foam, white with
foam;

Father toils amid the din;

But baby sleeps at home.

Hush the winds roar hoarse
and deep, —

On they come, on they come!

Brother seeks the wandering
sheep;

But baby sleeps at home.

Hush! the rain sweeps o'er
the knowes,

Where they roam, where
they roam;

Sister goes to seek the cows;

But baby sleeps at home.

Toys over Time

1900s
- Wind-up toys, Crayola crayons, teddy bears, jigsaw puzzles

1910s
- Raggedy Ann, Kewpie dolls

1920s
- Pogo sticks, the Duncan Yo-Yo, Mickey Mouse dolls, play doctor's bags

1930s
- The Viewmaster, Scrabble, Monopoly

1940s
- Slinkies, bubbles, rocking horses, paper dolls, dollhouses, Candy Land, Golden books, Dial typewriter

1950s
- Walkie-talkies, Yahtzee, toy telephones, Play-Doh, Barbie, Frisbee, Mr. Potato Head, Hula-Hoop, Chatty Cathy, Little People

1960s
- Easy-Bake Oven, Lite-Brite, Etch A Sketch, Lego, troll dolls, Twister

1970s
- Weebles, Magna Doodle, Hippity Hops, Spirograph, Talking Mattel-O-Phone, Charlie's Angels dolls, cassette radios

1980s
- My Little Pony, Cabbage Patch Kids, American Girl dolls, Strawberry Shortcake, Rainbow Brite

Old Maid

ard games are a good old-fashioned way to spend time together with your daughter and a great family tradition. Shuffle the deck and let the games begin!

Before you begin:

You'll need a deck of playing cards, and two or more players (three to four is best).

The goal:

To make pairs of all your cards and not be left with the single Queen, or Old Maid.

To play:

Remove one Queen from the deck of cards. This will leave an "Old Maid," or an unpaired Queen, in the deck.

Choose one player to be the dealer. The dealer shuffles the deck of cards and deals the cards clockwise to each player until they run out (it's okay if they aren't even).

Players should take inventory of their cards, removing all the pairs they have in their hand and putting them face-down in a pile in the center of the table.

The player to the left of the dealer (Player One) goes first by offering his or her cards to the player to their left (Player Two). Player One places his/her cards on the table face down and Player Two selects a card from them. Player Two will either make a pair to add to the pile, or add the unmatched card back into their hand.

The game continues this way, each player making pairs for all their cards. When a player has matched all the cards in their hand, they are safe, and when all the cards have been paired, whoever holds the remaining Queen is the Old Maid!

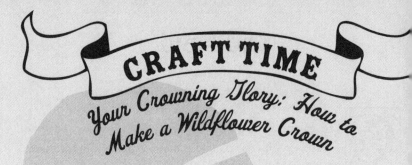

CRAFT TIME

Your Crowning Glory: How to Make a Wildflower Crown

Sometimes the simple things in life can be the most enjoyable. Your daughter will love exploring nature and finding the perfect flowers to create her very own wildflower crown.

What You'll Need:

➻ selection of pretty wildflowers (twenty to thirty) with soft stems at least four to five inches long, plus one or two "base" flowers with the longest stems (eight inches plus) to tie the other flowers to.

TO MAKE THE CROWN:

Lay your base flower(s) on a flat work surface, and knot the wildflowers and grasses around the stem of the base flower, twining and looping them around the base stem(s) a few times. Lay the excess stem of the wrapping flower parallel along the base flower's stem. Continue adding flowers and grasses to the base stems until you reach the desired length. Overlap the ends of the crown and tie them together using the stem pieces. Place the crown upon the Queen!

POEMS

The Owl and the Pussy-Cat

BY EDWARD LEAR

The Owl and the Pussy-Cat
went to sea

In a beautiful pea-green boat:

They took some honey, and
plenty of money

Wrapped up in a five-pound
note.

The Owl looked up to the
stars above,

And sang to a small guitar,

"O lovely Pussy, O Pussy,
my love,

What a beautiful Pussy you are,

You are,

You are!

What a beautiful Pussy you
are!"

Pussy said to the Owl, "You
elegant fowl,

How charmingly sweet you
sing!

Oh! let us be married; too long
we have tarried:

But what shall we do for a ring?"

They sailed away, for a year
and a day,

To the land where the bong-
tree grows;

And there in a wood a
Piggy-wig stood,

With a ring at the end of his nose,

His nose,

His nose,

With a ring at the end of his
nose.

"Dear Pig, are you willing to
sell for one shilling

Your ring?" Said the Piggy,
"I will."

So they took it away, and were
married next day

By the Turkey who lives
on the hill.

They dined on mince and
slices of quince,

Which they ate with a
runcible spoon;

And hand in hand, on the
edge of the sand.

They danced by the light
of the moon,

The moon,

The moon,

They danced by the light
of the moon.

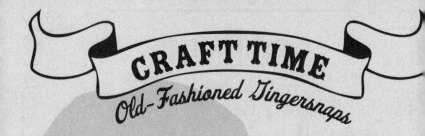

CRAFT TIME
Old-Fashioned Gingersnaps

These spicy cookies are both chewy and crisp. For a spicier cookie, add about ¼ teaspoon of cayenne pepper. It gives heat to the cinnamon without adding flavor.

Ingredients

YIELDS 36 COOKIES

- 2 teaspoons baking soda
- ¼ teaspoon salt
- 2 cups flour
- 1 teaspoon cinnamon
- 1 teaspoon ginger
- ¼ teaspoon cloves
- ¼ cup shortening
- ½ cup butter
- 1 cup sugar
- 1 cup unsulfured molasses
- 1 egg
- Sugar for rolling

1. Sift together baking soda, salt, flour, cinnamon, ginger, and cloves; set aside.

2. Cream shortening, butter, and 1 cup of sugar. Blend in molasses and egg.

3. Add dry ingredients to creamed mixture; blend well. Cover and chill 30 minutes or longer.

4. Preheat oven to 375°F. Butter baking sheets.

5. Shape dough into walnut-sized balls; roll in sugar. Place 2" apart on baking sheets; bake 12 minutes. Cool completely.

Little Red-Cap
(Little Red Riding Hood)

BY THE BROTHERS GRIMM

nce upon a time there was a dear little girl who was loved by everyone who looked at her, but most of all by her grandmother, and there was nothing that she would not have given to the child. Once she gave her a little cap of red velvet, which suited her so well that she would never wear anything else; so she was always called "Little Red-Cap."

One day her mother said to her: "Come, Little Red-Cap, here is a piece of cake and a bottle of wine; take them to your grandmother, she is ill and weak, and they will do her good. Set out before it gets hot, and when you are going, walk nicely and quietly and do not run off the path, or you may fall and break the bottle, and then your grandmother will get nothing; and when you go into her room, don't forget to say, 'Good morning,' and don't peep into every corner before you do it."

"I will take great care," said Little Red-Cap to her mother, and gave her hand on it.

The grandmother lived out in the wood, half a league from the village, and just as Little Red-Cap entered the wood, a wolf met her. Red-Cap did not know what a wicked creature he was, and was not at all afraid of him.

"Good day, Little Red-Cap," said he.

"Thank you kindly, wolf."

"Whither away so early, Little Red-Cap?"

"To my grandmother's."

"What have you got in your apron?"

"Cake and wine; yesterday was baking-day, so poor sick grand-mother is to have something good, to make her stronger."

"Where does your grandmother live, Little Red-Cap?"

"A good quarter of a league farther on in the wood; her house stands under the three large oak-trees, the nut-trees are just below; you surely must know it," replied Little Red-Cap.

The wolf thought to himself: "What a tender young creature! what a nice plump mouthful—she will be better to eat than the old woman. I must act craftily, so as to catch both." So he walked for a short time by the side of Little Red-Cap, and then he said: "See, Little Red-Cap, how pretty the flowers are about here—why do you not look round? I believe, too, that you do not hear how sweetly the little birds are singing; you walk gravely along as if you were going to school, while everything else out here in the wood is merry."

Little Red-Cap raised her eyes, and when she saw the sunbeams dancing here and there through the trees, and pretty flowers grow-ing everywhere, she thought: "Suppose I take grandmother a fresh nosegay; that would please her too. It is so early in the day that I shall still get there in good time"; and so she ran from the path into the wood to look for flowers. And whenever she had picked one, she fancied that she saw a still prettier one farther on, and ran after it, and so got deeper and deeper into the wood.

Meanwhile the wolf ran straight to the grandmother's house and knocked at the door.

"Who is there?"

"Little Red-Cap," replied the wolf. "She is bringing cake and wine; open the door."

"Lift the latch," called out the grandmother, "I am too weak, and cannot get up."

The wolf lifted the latch, the door sprang open, and without say-ing a word he went straight to the grandmother's bed, and devoured her. Then he put on her clothes, dressed himself in her cap laid himself in bed and drew the curtains.

Little Red-Cap, however, had been running about picking flowers, and when she had gathered so many that she could carry no more, she remembered her grandmother, and set out on the way to her.

She was surprised to find the cottage-door standing open, and when she went into the room, she had such a strange feeling that she said to herself: "Oh dear! how uneasy I feel today, and at other times I like being with grandmother so much." She called out: "Good morning," but received no answer; so she went to the bed and drew back the curtains. There lay her grandmother with her cap pulled far over her face, and looking very strange.

"Oh! grandmother," she said, "what big ears you have!"

"The better to hear you with, my child," was the reply.

"But, grandmother, what big eyes you have!" she said.

"The better to see you with, my dear."

"But, grandmother, what large hands you have!"

"The better to hug you with."

"Oh! but, grandmother, what a terrible big mouth you have!"

"The better to eat you with!"

And scarcely had the wolf said this, than with one bound he was out of bed and swallowed up Red-Cap.

When the wolf had appeased his appetite, he lay down again in the bed, fell asleep and began to snore very loud. The huntsman was just passing the house, and thought to himself: "How the old woman is snoring! I must just see if she wants anything." So he went into the room, and when he came to the bed, he saw that the wolf was lying in it. "Do I find you here, you old sinner!" said he. "I have long sought you!" Then just as he was going to fire at him, it occurred to him that the wolf might have devoured the grandmother, and that she might still be saved, so he did not fire, but took a pair of scissors, and began to cut open the stomach of the sleeping wolf. When he had made two snips, he saw the little Red-Cap shining, and then he made two snips more, and the little girl sprang out, crying: "Ah, how frightened I have been! How dark it was inside the wolf"; and after that the aged grandmother came out alive also, but scarcely able to breathe. Red-Cap, however, quickly fetched great stones with which they filled the wolf's belly, and when he awoke, he wanted to run away, but the stones were so heavy that he collapsed at once, and fell dead.

Then all three were delighted. The huntsman drew off the wolf's skin and went home with it; the grandmother ate the cake and drank the wine which Red-Cap had brought, and revived, but Red-Cap thought to herself: "As long as I live, I will never by myself leave the path, to run into the wood, when my mother has forbidden me to do so."

It also related that once when Red-Cap was again taking cakes to the old grandmother, another wolf spoke to her, and tried to entice her from the path. Red-Cap, however, was on her guard, and went straight forward on her way, and told her grandmother that she had met the wolf, and that he had said "good morning" to her, but with such a wicked look in his eyes, that if they had not been on the public road she was certain he would have eaten her up. "Well," said the grandmother, "we will shut the door, that he may not come in."

Soon afterwards the wolf knocked, and cried: "Open the door, grandmother, I am Little Red-Cap, and am bringing you some cakes." But they did not speak, or open the door, so the grey-beard stole twice or thrice round the house, and at last jumped on the roof, intending to wait until Red-Cap went home in the evening, and then to steal after her and devour her in the darkness. But the grandmother saw what was in his thoughts. In front of the house was a great stone trough, so she said to the child: "Take the pail,

Red-Cap; I made some sausages yesterday, so carry the water in which I boiled them to the trough." Red-Cap carried until the great trough was quite full. Then the smell of the sausages reached the wolf, and he sniffed and peeped down, and at last stretched out his neck so far that he could no longer keep his footing and began to slip, and slipped down from the roof straight into the great trough, and was drowned. But Red-Cap went joyously home, and no one ever did anything to harm her again.

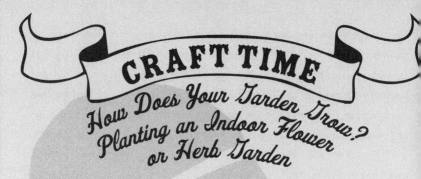

CRAFT TIME

How Does Your Garden Grow? Planting an Indoor Flower or Herb Garden

Learning about gardening is a great way to cultivate a love for nature in your daughter, and planting flowers or herbs is a great way to teach your growing daughter how to nurture and care for her garden as it grows.

What You'll Need:

First you'll need to decide what you'd like to plant together! These are some of the flowers and herbs that are easily grown indoors:

Flowers: Miniature roses, pansies, impatiens, dwarf sunflowers, nasturtiums, petunias, geraniums, marigolds

Herbs: Basil, parsley, chives, mint, lavender, oregano, rosemary, sage, thyme, tarragon

1. Next you'll need to find a container to plant your seeds in. A terra cotta pot works well, along with plastic or ceramic pots. But you can be as creative as you'd like. Old mugs, pots and pans, a sand pail, baskets (with a liner, of course), cookie jars, and coffee cans would all make for interesting planters! If you choose an unconventional container that you cannot make drainage holes in, add some rocks (or even marbles) in the bottom to provide drainage for the soil. Make sure there is something underneath your "pot" to catch any extra water.

2. Once you have your container, fill it with potting soil, leaving a few inches at the top. You can buy potting soil that is perfect for indoor planting at any garden center. Don't pack the soil in too tight, just give it a shake and let the soil settle in.

3. Now it's time to plant! Drop the seeds you've chosen on top of the soil, then cover with another ½" layer of earth.

4. Leave them to grow in a sunny window, remembering to water your flowers when the soil feels dry!

REFERENCE PAGE

Audet, Marye. *The Everything Cookies & Brownies Cookbook*. Avon, MA: Adams Media, 2009.

Fact Monster. "20th-Century Toys and Games Timeline." Last updated May 01, 2011. *www.factmonster.com/ipka/A0768872.html*.

The Holy Bible, New Living Translation (Illinois: Tyndale House Publishers, Inc., 2004).

How Stuff Works. "23 Must-Have Toys from the 1950s and Beyond" by the Editors of Publications International, Ltd., *http://entertainment.howstuffworks.com/23-must-have-toys-from-the-1950s-and-beyond.htm*. Accessed 19 March 2011.

Opie, I. and P. *The Oxford Dictionary of Nursery Rhymes*. 2nd edition. Oxford, UK: Oxford University Press, 1997.

Sheldon Vanauken, *A Severe Mercy* (New York: Harper Collins, 1980).

Social Security Administration. "Popular Baby Names by Decade." Last modified May 14, 2010. Social Security Online, *www.ssa.gov/oact/babynames/decades/index.html*.

Roberts, Dan. "The Best Selling Toys of the Last 50 Years." *www.dad.info/entertainment/books-toys-and-games/the-best-selling-toys-of-the-last-50-years*. Accessed 19 March 2011.

Toys Timeline, KPaul Media, *www.toystimeline.com*. Accessed 19 March 2011.

Andersen, Hans Christian. *Hans Andersen's Fairy Tales: First Series*. *www.gutenberg.org/ebooks/32571*. Accessed 11 May 2011.

Andersen, Hans Christian. *Hans Andersen's Fairy Tales: Second Series*. *www.gutenberg.org/ebooks/32572*. Accessed 11 May 2011.

Anonymous. "The Story of Goldilocks and the Three Bears." *www.dltk-teach.com/rhymes/goldilocks_story.htm*. Accessed 11 May 2011.

Greenaway, Kate. *Mother Goose or the Old Nursery Rhymes*. *www.gutenberg.org/ebooks/23794*. Accessed 23 May 2011.

Grimm, Jacob & Wilhelm. *Grimms' Fairy Tales*. *www.gutenberg.org/ebooks/2591*. Accessed 23 May 2011.

Grover, Eulalie Osgood (ed.). *Mother Goose: The Original Volland Edition*. *www.gutenberg.org/ebooks/24623*. Accessed 23 May 2011.

Lear, Edward. *Nonsense Books*. *www.gutenberg.org/ebooks/13650*. Accessed 23 May 2011.

Wright, Blanche Fisher. *The Real Mother Goose*. *www.gutenberg.org/ebooks/10607*. Accessed 23 May 2011.

About the Author

M. L. Stratton is a freelance editor who has been working in the publishing industry for over eight years. From editing presentations for worldwide IT conferences, to creating pamphlets for small non-profits, to blogging about her life at home, much of her world is wrapped up in words. On the off chance she's not chasing her three energetic kids around, you'll probably find her armed either with a book and a cup of tea, or a paintbrush and a pickaxe, working with her husband David to fix up her 163-year-old Cape.

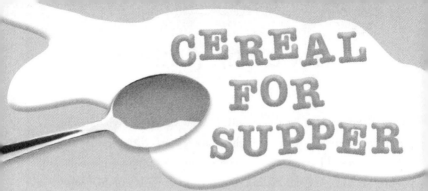

When You Don't Have Time for Anything Else

Visit our Cereal for Supper blog and join other over-inundated, under-celebrated, multi-tasking moms for an (almost) daily allowance of parenting advice—and absolution.

You won't learn how to make handmade Martha Stewart–inspired hankie holders or elaborate gourmet dinners—but you will find heaping spoonfuls of support and a few laughs along the way!

Sign up for our newsletter now at
www.adamsmedia.com/blog/parenting
And get our FREE Top Ten Recipes for Picky Eaters!